THE PREDIABETES DIET PLAN

How to Reverse Prediabetes
and Prevent Diabetes Through
Healthy Eating and Exercise

Hillary Wright, M.Ed, RD

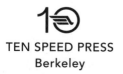

TEN SPEED PRESS
Berkeley

The illustrations herein are taken from *The PCOS Diet Plan* by Hillary Wright, published by Celestial Arts in 2010.

The Exchange Lists are the basis of a meal planning system designed by a committee of the American Diabetes Association and The American Dietetic Association. While designed primarily for people with diabetes and others who must follow special diets, the Exchange Lists are based on principles of good nutrition that apply to everyone. Copyright © 2008 by the American Diabetes Association and The American Dietetic Association.

Library of Congress Cataloging-in-Publication Data

Wright, Hillary.
  The prediabetes diet plan : how to reverse prediabetes and prevent diabetes through healthy eating and exercise / Hillary Wright, MEd, RD, LDN. — First edition.
      pages cm
1. Diabetes—Diet therapy. 2. Prediabetic state—Patients—Diet therapy.
3. Diabetes—Prevention. 4. Physical fitness. I. Title.
  RC662.W75 2013
  616.4'620654—dc23
                        2013018751

Trade Paperback ISBN: 978-1-60774-462-7
eBook ISBN: 978-1-60774-463-4

Printed in the United States of America

Design by Sarah Adelman

10 9 8 7 6 5 4 3 2 1

First Edition

Contents

Foreword

More than 26 million Americans have diabetes, so it's likely that you know someone with the condition, perhaps a family member or friend. Diabetes has serious health consequences, and it garners considerable attention from the medical community and the media. Prediabetes, the forerunner to diabetes, gets less press, but has recently come into its own and is being recognized as a force to be reckoned with.

While the number of Americans with diabetes is nothing to quibble about, more than three times as many people—an estimated 79 million—have prediabetes. With prediabetes, blood sugar (glucose) is higher than normal, but not yet elevated enough to be considered diabetes. Prediabetes may be symptom-free, and it's likely most people won't know that they have it until they take a blood test.

In spite of the somewhat disarming terminology, there's nothing "pre" about prediabetes, which, like diabetes, increases the risk of heart attack, stroke, and high blood pressure. Some experts argue that prediabetes and diabetes are actually one and the same condition, because harmful health effects from high blood sugar progress with time. In fact, about half of the people with prediabetes develop type 2 diabetes within ten years as their blood sugar levels creep upward.

The news isn't all bad, however. Today's prediabetes diagnosis need not become tomorrow's diabetes, nor does prediabetes necessarily have to play havoc with your health in any other way. There is hope for reversing prediabetes and preventing diabetes. That's the essence of *The Prediabetes Diet Plan*.

If you, or a loved one, have been advised to lower your blood sugar, you've come to the right book. Hillary Wright is a compassionate and experienced dietitian with an obvious passion for prevention. It will seem as though she is speaking directly to you in her warm, conversational tone when explaining the details of prediabetes and diabetes and how best to manage your health. As a highly skilled communicator, Hillary dishes up scientific evidence in easy-to-understand terms, an absolute must for understanding what's happening with your body.

Knowledge is power, but knowing what to do doesn't always mean you'll do it. As a registered dietitian who happens to have several relatives with type 2 diabetes, I am all too aware of how difficult it can be to change your eating habits, even when a better diet would greatly improve your health. *The Prediabetes Diet Plan* leaves no stone unturned on the topics of prediabetes and diabetes, but it also goes to great lengths to help you jumpstart your journey to better health and keep you, and the rest of your household, on the right path.

I especially appreciate the way Hillary avoids preaching about what you should do for better health. She goes out of her way to avoid giving one-size-fits-all advice about weight control, healthy eating, and blood sugar management. Hillary embraces difference, and, in that vein, presents reasonable, real-life scenarios to help guide lifestyle choices.

Consumers and health professionals alike should thank Hillary Wright for her laser focus on prediabetes, a condition that's become a personal burden for millions of Americans, as well as a financial strain on the health care system. Prediabetes, you're finally getting the attention you deserve!

Elizabeth M. Ward, MS, RD
Author, *MyPlate for Moms, How to Feed Yourself & Your Family Better*

Acknowledgments

As with any large undertaking, it took a village to guide and support me through this book. I'd like to start by thanking my parents, Alan and Marie Wright, who demonstrated that through education and strong family ties it's possible to raise healthy children with type 1 diabetes, and my brothers Michael and Christopher, and their families, who show every day that by taking care of yourself you can still live active, successful lives with this disease. To the rest of my siblings, Alison, John, and Brian, their families, my in-laws Jack and Nancy Holowitz, and the Holowitz/Parmentier clan, thank you all for your unwavering support.

To the hundreds of people with diabetes I have counseled and learned from over the years, thanks for teaching me the real challenges of living with this disease, and how taking small steps can make a difference. To my past, present, and future patients with prediabetes, including all my "PCOS girls," this one's for you.

Thanks to my agent, Judith Riven, my editor, Sara Golski, all the folks at Ten Speed Press, dietetic intern Emma Laskey, and graphic artist David Parmentier for helping to massage this book into its final form. Also, the encouragement of my friends and colleagues at the Domar Center for Mind/Body Health and the Dana Farber Cancer Institute has been invaluable.

On a personal level, words can't express how much I valued the support of my "townie" friends, my fabulous nutrition pals, and my nutrition "soul mate," Elizabeth Ward, MS, RD, during this crazy time. Most importantly, thanks so much to Tony, John, Matt, and Brian. Without your love and ability to laugh with and at me, none of this would have come to be. I love you.

Introduction

Talk about diabetes is everywhere—on the nightly news, in health magazines, and most definitely in the doctor's office. In my world, it seems like the subject has always been present. I'm one of six children, and when I was twelve, my seven-year-old brother was diagnosed with type 1 diabetes. At the time all I understood was that he had to take shots of insulin every day. If he took too much, it could kill him, so he always had to carry a snack. It was pretty scary stuff for us kids, but my parents were so proactive about learning how to manage my brother's condition that before long, it was just part of our family's reality. My mother credits a dietitian at Children's Hospital in Boston with helping them feel confident in their ability to manage my brother's diabetes. (This woman, by the way, was also the inspiration for my mother to encourage me to become a dietitian.)

Several years later, when my youngest brother was eleven, he too was diagnosed with type 1 diabetes. Although I'm sure this second diagnosis was devastating for my parents, by this point the rest of us were pretty used to what would be involved. Back in those days, it seemed unique to have two siblings with diabetes, but because my parents had learned what they needed to manage my brothers' health, both brothers, now in their forties, are happy, healthy, and busy with their own families and careers. Not everyone who develops diabetes this young is as lucky, however. Early-onset diabetes (either type 1 or type 2 diagnosed early in life) is associated with a host of health complications, including heart disease, kidney failure, and blindness. Type 1 diabetes accounts for about 10 percent of all diabetes. Because injected insulin is necessary to manage the disease, type 1 diabetes requires intensive day-to-day attention to stay safe and healthy. The other 90 percent of diabetes is type 2 diabetes, which was once referred to as "adult onset" because it almost always affected adults, but now unfortunately is also affecting children due to the escalating rates of childhood obesity.

When I began my career as a hospital nutritionist in the late 1980s, I learned to associate type 2 diabetes with complications. Back then, many of my patients had not been routinely screened for diabetes (as they are more likely to be today). In fact, many of them did not even know they were diabetic until they went to the eye doctor complaining of vision problems, only to find out they were suffering from diabetic retinopathy (a common cause of blindness). This complication would suggest that they had been walking around with diabetes for years, maybe even decades, without knowing it. Many of them suffered from severe forms of vascular disease. In fact, about 65 percent of people with diabetes die of heart disease or stroke.[1] Caring for so many people with diabetes—a serious, largely preventable illness—was discouraging. Even more depressing, many of them hadn't had the chance to avoid the poor health that eventually befell them because they didn't even know they had diabetes!

There's no guarantee that someone with knowledge of a health problem is ready, willing, or able to do something about it, and the more years that pass without trying to change one's habits can make it increasingly harder to eventually get there. Dietitians know that nutrition education during hospitalization isn't the ideal time or setting to teach people how to eat differently or change their lifestyle—there are generally too many other more acute health issues to focus on—but I did my best during these years to help my patients see that even small changes could make a difference. Given the readmission rates of my diabetic patients, however, I saw firsthand that trying to help them eat healthier and get a little exercise through my in-hospital education sessions was like swimming upstream.

So after six years of hospital work, I decided to put my counseling skills to work in the area of prevention. By this time, I had several relatives with type 2 diabetes who were taking good care of themselves and staying healthy. I understood that diabetes was something to tackle early on—even before diagnosis. What we appreciate now more than we did twenty years ago is that *diabetes can be prevented!* According to data on almost eighty-five thousand women from the Harvard Nurse's Health study, about 90 percent of type 2 diabetes cases in women can be attributed to such lifestyle factors as excess weight, lack of exercise, a less-than-healthy diet, and smoking, and there's no reason the same shouldn't be true of men.[2] Preventing diabetes might be easier than many people think. According to the American Diabetes Association, studies have shown that type 2 diabetes may be prevented or delayed by losing just

7 percent of one's body weight (for example, this is just fifteen pounds for a two-hundred-pound person) through regular physical activity (thirty minutes a day, five days a week) and healthy eating.[3] For most people, making changes to their diet and lifestyle is not easy. Uprooting old habits and replacing them with healthier ones is tough. The process takes time. Readiness to make these important changes is a strong predictor of success, and no one can make someone else be "ready." Rather, readiness has to come from within. Concern about a new health threat—in oneself or a close family member or friend—can often move someone closer to readiness to make important diet and lifestyle changes. Primary care doctors today are much more likely to screen for diabetes earlier in life—even in children—so increasingly people are learning that they are at risk for developing diabetes (based on medical or family history). In some cases, people discover that they are actually already prediabetic. This means that their blood sugar levels are starting to rise but are not yet high enough to be classified as diabetes.

In a perfect world, we'd all know what our risk is and be able to address it *before* prediabetes sets in. It would be ideal to avoid having problems with blood glucose regulation by addressing it prior to the point when you start flunking your blood glucose tests. The reality is, however, that sometimes we need to see it in black-and-white on a lab slip: that fasting blood glucose test with an H (for "high") next to it. For many people, this isn't surprising news, particularly if they've been overweight for a long time or if there is a lot of diabetes in the family. My hope is that, armed with the knowledge that type 2 diabetes is something that can be prevented, people will use this health threat as the starting gate to get into the game of diabetes prevention.

As a registered dietitian with more than two decades of experience helping people manage their diabetes, I've counseled thousands of men and women from all walks of life on how to start with their current habits and move toward a healthier place. Since 2000, I've also been counseling women with an endocrine problem called polycystic ovary syndrome (PCOS), which is a major cause of infertility and places women with the condition in a high-risk category for type 2 diabetes. While no one would want a condition like PCOS (which also increases the risk of cardiovascular disease), at least these women know they are at higher risk of developing diabetes and are often motivated to learn how to reduce their risk. The same diet and lifestyle strategies that can improve their fertility also lower their risk of diabetes. In 2010, I wrote a book on diet and lifestyle management of PCOS, *The PCOS Diet Plan*. The idea for *The Prediabetes Diet Plan* came from a physician, Dr. Diane Kaufman, who told me she advises all her patients with prediabetes to read *The PCOS Diet Plan* "and just skip over the PCOS parts."

There is an urgent need for more information on managing prediabetes through a healthy diet and lifestyle. Applying what I know about managing insulin resistance—the condition that underlies both prediabetes and PCOS—I focus in this book on diabetes prevention. My goal is to provide the same sense of empowerment and doable, realistic diet and lifestyle strategies to the much larger population of people who have prediabetes. To support the positive thinking needed to allow for change, I interject "Mind-Set Interventions" throughout the book. I can't emphasize enough how important it is to pay as much—or more—attention to what's going on with your mind as with your grocery cart, your lunch choice, or your exercise options. Positive, healthy diet and lifestyle changes have to start between your ears long before they have a chance to change what's happening in your body.

A final thought on what this book isn't: it's not a diabetes book. A book that tries to deal with both diabetes prevention and diabetes management has the potential to try to do too much for too many people with varying needs. There are many excellent books written by talented registered dietitians for those who already have diabetes (several of these are listed in the Resources section in the back of the book). The goal of *The Prediabetes Diet Plan* is to reduce the number of people who need resources for diabetes—or at a minimum, to delay that need for as long as possible. As I tell my patients, I'm like the tugboat that's there to drag you out of the harbor so you can sail on your own. I have no preconception of how long, or what path, that process takes. The journey is different for everyone. By sharing some useful strategies—and encouraging you to view lapses not as failures but as opportunities to learn—you'll soon find yourself charting a course to better health.

Part 1

DEFINING PREDIABETES AND ITS CAUSES

1

Understanding Prediabetes

"Prediabetes" refers to the phase before a person develops diabetes, where blood glucose levels are higher than normal but not high enough for the person to be diagnosed with diabetes. To really understand that definition, you need to first know what diabetes is and what you are trying to avoid. According to the Centers for Disease Control (CDC), rates of type 2 diabetes have more than tripled in the United States since the early 1990s, fueled largely by the global obesity epidemic.[1] Most people know that diabetes is when you have too much sugar in your blood—"sugar" here referring to blood glucose, which is the body's fuel ("blood glucose" is the technical term and "blood sugar" is the layperson's term). In my experience, though, most people with diabetes don't have a complete or even adequate understanding of what's happening in their bodies when they have this disease. This lack of understanding makes it tough to internalize what they need to do to manage the condition. This knowledge deficit is undoubtedly more significant in the much larger numbers of people who have prediabetes—most of whom don't know it.

Diabetes: A Simple Explanation

Diabetes is a chronic medical condition in which the body has a reduced ability to clear glucose out of the blood and into the body's cells after eating or drinking anything that contains carbohydrates. This reduced ability results in elevated blood glucose, or hyperglycemia. Type 2 diabetes is caused by the coexistence over time of two conditions: insulin resistance and chronic inflammation. This results in a progressive state where the body needs to produce higher than normal amounts of the hormone insulin to clear glucose out of the blood after a meal or snack that contains carbohydrates. Insulin resistance starts at a low or "subclinical" level that can exist for years before being diagnosed by a blood test. If left untreated, however, glucose levels can worsen over time (particularly right after meals) until eventually a fasting blood glucose test shows elevation— clear evidence that someone is potentially progressing from prediabetes toward full-blown diabetes. Insulin resistance occurs on a spectrum: it starts at a low level, where there's no easy test to see that it's happening; as it progresses, insulin resistance eventually shows up as prediabetes; and if not addressed through diet, lifestyle change, and possibly medication, insulin resistance may progress further to diabetes.

Current estimates are that most individuals with prediabetes—possibly as many as 70 percent—will eventually develop type 2 diabetes.[2] Aside from high blood glucose levels, diabetes is associated with a host of other health problems, including heart disease, stroke, amputations, kidney failure, cancer, and cognitive (brain function) problems. Research tells us that the risk of all these problems can be greatly reduced, or even avoided altogether, when healthy lifestyle changes are implemented early on. As the old saying goes, an ounce of prevention is worth a pound of cure!

Don't worry if this explanation about insulin resistance, prediabetes, and diabetes doesn't yet make much sense. We'll review throughout the book how this process might play out in an individual moving through this progression. By the time someone is diagnosed with diabetes, insulin resistance has been present for some time (probably years) and has progressed through a stage where the individual was—or could have been—diagnosed with prediabetes. Not everyone who is diagnosed with prediabetes will go on to develop type 2 diabetes, but its presence puts one in a higher risk category for the development of diabetes. Managing insulin resistance to treat prediabetes, and possibly prevent it from progressing to type 2 diabetes, is what this book is all about. You'll learn how to determine whether you may have prediabetes and what you can do to avoid or delay its progression to diabetes. Unfortunately, once someone has diabetes, it can't be cured (the condition can only be controlled by weight loss or various interventions), whereas prediabetes can often be reversed. These are very important distinctions between prediabetes and diabetes.

Elevated blood glucose is generally without symptoms until it gets very high (at levels you would experience only if you were already diabetic and your glucose levels were way out of control). Just because you don't feel anything doesn't mean it isn't there. In a way it's unfortunate that hyperglycemia doesn't hurt a little because people would be more aware that something is wrong and might be compelled to pay attention to it. Despite its lack of symptoms in the early stages, diabetes is a serious problem with potentially very serious consequences. Before we move on to the must-know information on diabetes and prediabetes, let's start with some facts about how these conditions have affected the health and wellness of people in the United States.

Alarming Statistics in the United States

According to 2011 data from the American Diabetes Association, the number of people affected by diabetes and prediabetes is enormous and getting larger.[3] Consider these statistics:

- The total prevalence of diabetes in the United States is 25.8 million children and adults, or 8.3 percent of the population. There are 18.8 million diagnosed cases of diabetes in the United States and an estimated 7 million undiagnosed cases. The number of diagnosed cases has more than tripled since 1980, when the number of Americans diagnosed with diabetes was 5.6 million.[4]
- The number of children and adolescents with diabetes: 1 in 400.
- The number of people age sixty-five and older with diabetes: 10.9 million, or 26.9 percent of all people in this age group.
- The estimated number of people in the United States with prediabetes is a whopping 79 million. Thirty-five percent of US adults age twenty and older and 50 percent of those age sixty-five and older are prediabetic.[5]

Diabetes is an equal opportunity disease, affecting both men and women in the United States:

- 13 million men, or 11.8 percent of all men age twenty and older, have diabetes.
- 12.6 million women, or 10.8 percent of all women age twenty and older, have diabetes.

The disease doesn't discriminate by race and ethnicity either. Here's a breakdown by race and ethnicity of people ages twenty and older diagnosed with diabetes:

- 7.1 percent of non-Hispanic whites
- 8.4 percent of Asian Americans
- 12.6 percent of non-Hispanic blacks
- 11.8 percent of Hispanics

And things don't look good for the future health of US children. According to the CDC, if current trends continue, one in three children born in 2000 will develop diabetes in their lifetimes.[6]

Diabetes is a major cause of morbidity and mortality in the United States. In 2007 the disease contributed to 231,404 deaths. What makes diabetes so potentially life threatening is the close association between diabetes and serious health problems such as heart disease, stroke, high blood pressure, and cancer. Consider these sobering facts: In 2004 heart disease was noted as the cause of death in 68 percent of diabetics age sixty-five and older (adults with diabetes have heart disease death rates two to four times higher than adults without diabetes). In 2004 stroke was noted as the cause of death in 16 percent of diabetics age sixty-five and older (risk of stroke is two to four times higher among people with diabetes). During the period 2005 to 2008, of adults age twenty and older with self-reported diabetes, 67 percent had high blood pressure or used prescription drugs for hypertension.

The impact of diabetes on quality of life is enormous. Diabetes is a leading cause of blindness, kidney failure, neuropathy (a painful condition caused by damage to the tiny blood vessels that nourish nerve cells, particularly in the legs), and lower-limb amputations (again, due to blood vessel damage over time). As you can imagine, the price tag that goes along with treating diabetes and its complications is huge, and on track to get a lot bigger: In 2012 the total cost of diagnosed diabetes in the United States was $245 billion ($176 billion for medical costs and $69 billion for indirect costs associated with disability, lost work, and premature death). This represents a 41 percent increase since these costs were last estimated in 2007 (at $174 million dollars).[7] Adjusting for population age and sex differences, average medical expenditures for people diagnosed with diabetes were 2.3 times higher than for those without diabetes. Overall, the economic cost of dealing with diabetes is about a third of what was budgeted on national defense in 2012![8]

What's the bottom line? If there was ever a disease to avoid—for life expectancy and personal quality of life, as well as for the current and future economic health of the United States—diabetes is it. The good news is that we know a lot about how to prevent this disease. Research has proven that type 2 diabetes may be entirely avoidable! If you're prediabetic, the time to act is now. Currently about one in ten US adults has diabetes, and statistical trends suggest that by 2050 the incidence may be as high as one in three.[9] By learning to manage the underlying physiology that causes prediabetes (and subsequently diabetes)—insulin resistance—diabetes can be prevented. Prediabetes can be cured. The first step is determining if your family history or lifestyle places you at higher risk.

Causes of Prediabetes and Diabetes: Nature or Nurture?

As you look within your family, you may wonder whether diabetes is a genetic condition. Research suggests the genetics of type 2 diabetes is complex and that some people may have a strong genetic predisposition to it. In many people, however, risk can also be influenced by environmental and behavioral factors, like obesity and a sedentary lifestyle, on some underlying susceptibility that isn't yet fully understood.[10] It's often difficult to determine whether diabetes appears to be running in families because of a genetic predisposition or because of an "inheritance" of unhealthful diet and lifestyle habits that have been passed down from one generation to another. One interesting aspect to the diabetes epidemic is the theory that physiological factors currently predisposing people to diabetes may actually have been a survival adaptation that was at one time beneficial. Some scientists believe that insulin resistance is a genetically predetermined physiological trait, a so-called thrifty gene, that helped our primitive ancestors survive under conditions of drought and famine, and is now backfiring under modern lifestyle conditions where obesity and physical inactivity are common.[11] In other words, it's a "good gene gone bad" scenario.

There is a lot we still don't understand about why this harmful state is so common today, but this theory lends credence to the concept that the best way to counter any physiological predisposition to diabetes is to evolve your lifestyle to one better suited to our caveman makeup. While you can't control the genes you were born with, type 2 diabetes is largely a preventable disease (up to 90 percent of cases may be attributable to lifestyle habits), and a number of lifestyle risk factors can potently increase your risk for developing it.[12] Unfortunately, every one of these risk factors, summarized below, is common in our modern environment:

- **Obesity.** Obesity and weight gain dramatically increase the risk of type 2 diabetes and are considered the strongest contributors to the explosion of this disease in the US population.
- **Physical inactivity.** Independent of whether someone is overweight or obese, physical inactivity increases diabetes risk.
- **Cigarette smoking.** This habit is associated with a small increased risk of diabetes.
- **Low fiber diet.** Eating a diet low in fiber and high in processed foods increases risk.[13]
- **Saturated fats.** Results of human studies are mixed, but according to the *Archives of Internal Medicine*, studies suggest that diets high in saturated fats may worsen insulin resistance and increase diabetes risk.[14]
- **Sugar-sweetened beverages.** Regular consumption of these beverages has been shown to increase type 2 diabetes risk.

Factors That Increase Diabetes Risk

It's one thing to know that something may be increasing your risk of developing diabetes, but in my experience, understanding *why* helps a lot of people visualize the value of nudging these risk factors out of one's life. Let's look at the unhealthy influence of each risk factor in more detail.

Obesity

According to the National Institute of Diabetes and Digestive and Kidney Diseases, about 80 percent of people with type 2 diabetes are overweight or obese.[15] How obesity contributes to diabetes is complex and involves multiple influences, but research has identified the following factors as playing a significant role:

- Fat cells secrete fatty acids that contribute to insulin resistance in the liver and muscles of obese people.
- Fat cells secrete a large number of proteins that affect glucose ("blood sugar") metabolism and insulin action.
- Obesity increases inflammation in the body, which is closely tied to diabetes.

The physiological stress of obesity on the body seems to worsen insulin resistance in the cells and may reduce the pancreas's ability to secrete enough extra insulin to overcome this resistance, which leads to higher blood sugars.[16] Obesity often goes hand in hand with many of the other risk factors for diabetes, like physical inactivity and a low-fiber diet.

Physical Inactivity

According to the *Archives of Internal Medicine*, a significant body of research has shown that physical inactivity increases your risk of diabetes regardless of whether you're overweight or obese. Conversely, if you *are* overweight or obese, being physically active is one of the most helpful things you can do to naturally lower your diabetes risk.[17] Physical activity doesn't need to be vigorous to affect diabetes risk. One large analysis of ten studies, published in *Diabetes Care*, found that regular participation in moderately intense activity (like daily walking for thirty minutes or longer) substantially lowers the risk, even if you don't lose weight.[18] Physical activity increases insulin and glucose absorption into muscle (that is, it improves insulin sensitivity), whether baseline levels of glucose are normal or elevated (called impaired glucose tolerance), making it a key strategy for diabetes prevention in someone with prediabetes. Physical activity seems to be particularly helpful for reducing abdominal (belly) fat, which is known to aggravate insulin resistance and contribute to other health problems, such as high blood pressure and high triglycerides, that can raise your risk of heart disease.[19] Physical activity is also an important component of any weight-loss program.

Cigarette Smoking

Smokers are at higher risk of diabetes than nonsmokers, possibly because of the increased inflammation that cigarette smoke causes in the body.[20] Smoking has been shown to cause elevations in blood glucose levels and may worsen insulin resistance. Smokers tend to have more abdominal fat, also associated with insulin resistance.[21]

Low Fiber Diet

Dietary fiber does not raise blood glucose levels because it is not broken down in our digestive tracts. Eating high fiber foods will therefore decrease the amount of insulin needed after a meal or snack. High-fiber diets may also help with weight control. Cereal fiber in particular has been tied to lower likelihood of developing diabetes.[22] The American Diabetes Association recommends 25 to 30 grams of fiber each day, though it acknowledges that most of us only get about half of this recommended amount, so any increase in dietary fiber would be beneficial.[23]

Saturated Fats

Research suggests a link between dietary saturated fat and risk of diabetes. According to the US Department of Agriculture (USDA) Nutrition Evidence Library, replacing some saturated fat in the diet with heart-healthy fats (such as olive or canola oil, nuts, and avocados) may improve insulin resistance.[24] Other research in the journal *Nature Immunology* suggests that saturated fats may spur inflammation in liver, muscle, and fat cells, making them insulin resistant.[25] Some research points toward unhealthy trans fats as possibly having a similar effect, but evidence is limited.

Sugar-Sweetened Beverages

A huge 2010 analysis of eleven studies, including 310,819 participants and 15,043 cases of type 2 diabetes, found that those who consumed as little as one to two sugar-sweetened beverages a day had a 26 percent greater risk of developing type 2 diabetes than those who reported drinking fewer than one soda a month.[26] Sugar-sweetened beverages include soda, fruit-flavored drinks, sweetened iced tea, and so-called energy drinks. Sugar-sweetened beverages may contribute to the risk of type 2 diabetes in several ways: they are a commonly consumed source of excess calories (contributing to obesity); they provide a large load of easily absorbed carbs that spike blood glucose levels and tax the pancreas's ability to produce enough insulin to clear it; and they are a possible source of additional additives that may aggravate insulin resistance.[27] Fortunately, diet soda does not seem to carry the same risks but is worth consuming in moderation due to other potential health concerns, including some suspicion these drinks may increase people's subsequent cravings for highly sweetened foods.[28]

The common thread through all of these very prevalent modern lifestyle habits or unhealthy situations is that, one way or another, they contribute to the physiologically dangerous condition of insulin resistance. As mentioned earlier, humans may have evolved to become insulin resistant as part of a survival strategy. This trait may have helped us avoid starvation during times of drought and famine by redistributing our energy metabolism to give the body's vital cells a fair shot at glucose, the body's life-sustaining energy source. Likewise, pregnancy hormones trigger insulin resistance in pregnant women as a means of diverting glucose from the mother's cells to those of her developing baby to fuel rapid growth (hence the increased risk of gestational, or pregnancy-induced, diabetes in women who are already somewhat insulin resistant). In short, insulin resistance may have been incredibly important to the survival of our species but now stands to threaten it.

Other Insulin-Resistant Conditions: Metabolic Syndrome and PCOS

Even if you don't have prediabetes or diabetes, insulin resistance could be threatening your health by contributing to other increasingly common health problems. Although the focus of this book is treating prediabetes, there are two other common conditions in which insulin resistance is a major player: metabolic syndrome and polycystic ovary syndrome (PCOS). Both are considered major risk factors for the development of diabetes. Let's learn a bit more about each condition.

Metabolic Syndrome

This common and complex health condition is skyrocketing in the US population and contributing to the epidemic of diabetes and heart disease in a major way. About 35 percent of US adults have metabolic syndrome, which is driven by insulin resistance and chronic inflammation and is characterized by a collection of cardiovascular risk factors. An estimated 87 percent of those with diabetes also classify as having metabolic syndrome.[29] According to the American Heart Association, metabolic syndrome occurs when a person has three or more of the following measurements:

- Abdominal obesity (excessive belly fat)
- Triglyceride level of 150 milligrams per deciliter of blood (mg/dl) or greater
- HDL cholesterol level of less than 40 mg/dl in men or less than 50 mg/dl in women
- Systolic blood pressure (the top number) of 130 millimeters of mercury (mmHg) or greater
- Diastolic blood pressure (the bottom number) of 85 mmHg or greater
- Fasting glucose of 100 mg/dl or greater
- Insulin resistance or glucose intolerance[30]

Although this may vary by race, excess belly fat is generally defined as a waist circumference of 40 inches (102 centimeters) or more for men and 35 inches (88 centimeters) or more for women.[31] People with metabolic syndrome also have a tendency for their blood to clot more easily (called a prothrombic state), and they are more likely to have chronic inflammation in their bodies (called a proinflammatory state, which can be diagnosed with a C-reactive protein test, a marker for inflammation in the blood). Both of these conditions are like lighter fluid on the fire of heart disease risk. Although any of these factors can increase your risk of having a heart attack—and individually each risk factor should be treated aggressively—when present together, as in metabolic syndrome, the risk of having cardiovascular problems is significantly greater.[32] A recent review of the research on metabolic syndrome found that, overall, metabolic syndrome doubled the risk of cardiovascular disease, heart attack, and stroke and increased the chance of dying from any cause by 50 percent.[33]

Some ethnic groups are more affected by metabolic syndrome than others, with Mexican Americans having the highest rates, followed by whites and African Americans. Among Mexican Americans and African

Americans, metabolic syndrome is more common in women than men, but the syndrome affects white men and women about equally.[34] Despite having less body fat on average than whites, Asian Americans have higher rates of metabolic syndrome and diabetes, with both conditions growing rapidly among Asians and Pacific Islanders who have immigrated to the United States.[35] Research published in *Diabetes Care* suggests that Asians have more body fat at a lower BMI (body mass index) than whites and that people of Chinese descent have a similar risk of glucose intolerance at a lower BMI than people of European descent.[36] Although research is ongoing, it is believed that the combination of consuming a Western diet high in fat and calories, decreased physical activity, and genetic make-up is fueling this metabolic syndrome/diabetes epidemic in Asian populations in the United States.[37] Others at risk of metabolic syndrome include the following:

- Those who have a sibling or parent with diabetes
- Those who already have diabetes
- Women with PCOS

Polycystic Ovary Syndrome

This strange-sounding syndrome is the most common hormonal disorder of women in their reproductive years, affecting 5 to 10 percent (possibly more) of all women, and is the main cause of infertility related to irregular or absent ovulation. Research suggests that up to 30 percent of women have some of the symptoms of the disorder. And with the dramatic increase in childhood obesity, which often leads to earlier-onset menstruation, PCOS is already starting to show up in younger girls. Increasingly, PCOS has been recognized as being a major risk factor for prediabetes, diabetes, and heart disease. Like metabolic syndrome, PCOS is a complex problem, but it is believed that insulin resistance is a significant player in at least 75 percent of cases. In this scenario the elevated insulin levels, present because of underlying insulin resistance, interfere with the exquisite hormonal balance needed to trigger ovulation, leading to trouble conceiving. Insulin is a hormone, and as such has the ability to interfere with other circulating hormones. In PCOS this can trigger reproductive hormone imbalances that spawn some of the secondary symptoms of the condition, including excess levels of androgens, or male-type hormones, that cause abnormal hair growth on the face and other areas on the body.

As with insulin resistance from any cause, the strain on the pancreas to make extra insulin over time can wear down its ability to produce enough, leading to elevated glucose levels and prediabetes. Research suggests more than 50 percent of women with PCOS will have diabetes or prediabetes before the age of forty.[38] The cause of PCOS is not understood, but it is believed to be a complex genetic disorder likely involving multiple genes. Genes involved may be those that regulate function of the hypothalamus, pituitary, and ovaries, as well as those responsible for insulin resistance. Women with PCOS experience similar risk for the development of metabolic and cardiovascular problems as those diagnosed with metabolic syndrome, which makes sense given that in both conditions insulin resistance is a contributing factor.[39]

Anywhere from 50 to 80 percent of women with PCOS are overweight or obese, and the incidence of PCOS in the US population has paralleled the increase in obesity, suggesting a strong connection between body weight and the severity of the condition. Because hormone imbalance is a major side effect of PCOS, many of the symptoms are hormone related. Physical signs that a woman's hormone levels may be out of whack due to PCOS include the following:

- Infrequent or absent menstrual periods (signaling problems with ovulation)
- Excess hair growth on the face, chest, and back in a male pattern
- Thinning of the hair on the crown of the head
- Acne
- A tendency to accrue belly fat, or the "apple body" form of fat storage (as opposed to the healthier "pear," who stores her body fat more in the butt and thighs)

Women with PCOS are more likely to have elevated blood glucose levels as well as high blood cholesterol and triglyceride (blood fats) levels, along with low levels of healthy HDL cholesterol at a young age.

The Dangers of Insulin Resistance

What prediabetes, metabolic syndrome, and PCOS have in common is insulin resistance, which even without it having progressed to diabetes is a hazard to your cardiovascular system, and potentially to other organs. Although we have established cutoffs for diagnosing diabetes and prediabetes, insulin resistance is present even before any tests show signs of its presence, and it may already be wreaking havoc with your circulatory system. We know that many people with prediabetes also qualify as having metabolic syndrome. Most people with prediabetes and metabolic syndrome are also obese, which increases circulating levels of fats (triglycerides) and other substances that contribute to inflammation in the blood vessels and make the blood more likely to form clots, which can in turn clog arteries and cause a heart attack. These excess circulating fats can aggravate insulin resistance in the muscle, contributing to high blood glucose levels and lower healthy HDL levels.

Insulin resistance alone is known to be an independent risk factor for cardiovascular disease as it is believed to affect the health of the endothelium, or lining of the blood vessels, in several ways. Injury to the endothelium is considered the initiating factor in the development of cholesterol blockages in the arteries. Just the presence of higher-than-healthy levels of glucose, even if lower than that needed for a diagnosis of diabetes, have been reported to cause damage to the insides of blood vessels. There is a lot of crossover between metabolic syndrome and prediabetes, which can make it complicated for scientists to determine what is causing what when it comes to heart disease. Having metabolic syndrome alone without prediabetes (meaning a fasting blood glucose of 100 milligrams per deciliter or higher is *not* one of your three qualifiers from the metabolic syndrome list) raises your risk of diabetes fivefold. Having both prediabetes and metabolic syndrome raises your risk of diabetes even further. There is no predetermined blood glucose cutoff at which microvascular changes (meaning damage to the very smallest branches of the arteries that feed blood to the body's tissues) can start to occur. Some research suggests that prediabetes is associated with a small but appreciable increased risk for diabetic retinopathy, nephropathy (microscopic changes to the health of the kidneys), and neuropathy.[40]

Prediabetes is also thought to possibly affect brain health, contributing to premature aging of the brain and Alzheimer's disease.[41]

A person can start developing the typical diabetes complications in the prediabetic phase of the disease because it appears that the unhealthy effect of high blood sugar occurs on a continuum—it may start when the problem is in its early stages and worsen as the blood glucose levels get higher over time. Although more needs to be learned about how intervening earlier in the process may change the course of things, the hope is that lowering blood glucose levels to normal by treating insulin resistance early can help reduce any risk of damage to the large circulation—like the large arteries that feed the heart—as well as the microcirculation that keeps our eyes (retina), kidneys, and nerves healthy. Recent scientific evidence has also begun to tie insulin resistance to increased risk of a number of cancers, including cancer of the colon, liver, pancreas, and breast. The mechanisms for this connection aren't fully understood yet, but the following factors may play a role:

- High levels of glucose and insulin promote the release of insulin-like growth factor I (IGF-I), which may play a role in tumor initiation and progression in those who are insulin resistant.
- Higher levels of insulin and IGF-I inhibit the production of a protein that is supposed to bind with sex hormones (like estrogen and testosterone) and make them less available to encourage the growth of cancer in breast and endometrial (uterine) tissue.
- Insulin-resistant people may overproduce free radicals due to excessive oxidation, which may damage cell DNA and increase the likelihood they may mutate into cancer.
- The coexistence of obesity and insulin resistance may increase inflammation in the body, creating an environment that is conducive to the growth of tumors.[42]

In some ways this connection isn't new, as type 2 diabetes is known to significantly increase the risk of many forms of cancer because of the way it changes the body's physiological environment.[43] But just as insulin resistance may contribute to cancer risk, making changes to manage it can lower your risk. This is treatable and reversible.

What Is Inflammation?

Inflammation is a natural part of healing, but is meant to emerge as needed, then disappear. In contemporary times, however, a host of irritants (like smoking, obesity, inactivity, and excess intake of too much processed food) can lead to chronic, low-grade inflammation that sticks around. This can fuel the development of heart disease, diabetes (by aggravating insulin resistance), cancer, and other chronic diseases. Inflammation can be reduced by achieving a healthy weight, exercising, and eating a diet high in plant foods and heart-healthy fats (like vegetable oils, nuts, and seeds) and low in sugar and processed foods. Vitamin D and omega-3 fatty acids from seafood, vegetable oils, walnuts, and flax are also anti-inflammatory.

Helpful, Hopeful Information

Despite the statistics, not all the news is bad! There are many reasons to be optimistic. Even if you've already been diagnosed with prediabetes, it's possible it can be reversed. The odds of progressing to diabetes are high without investing a lot of time and energy into changing the unhealthful diet and lifestyle habits that may have gotten you to this point. But type 2 diabetes is a largely preventable disease, and treating it at the prediabetes phase—or sooner, if you know you're at risk—is hands down the best approach. Adopting healthful diet and lifestyle changes will likely improve your daily quality of life in many ways and may lower your risk of developing diabetes by up to 89 percent! But the solution isn't just making single behavior changes, like avoiding sugar, for example. Rather, you must address a collection of poor lifestyle habits. Each one of these contributes to an individual's risk of diabetes, and the more unhealthful habits you've acquired, the more your risk of prediabetes and diabetes mounts. Fortunately, the reverse is also true: the more unhealthy habits you replace with healthier ones, the lower your risk.

One very large 2009 study of almost five thousand men and women age sixty-five and older enrolled in the Cardiovascular Health Study looked at the participants' diet and lifestyle habits, along with whether or not they developed diabetes over a ten-year period. Low-risk diet and lifestyle behaviors identified among the participants were the following:

- Above-average physical activity levels
- Higher dietary fiber intake

- Eating more heart-healthy polyunsaturated fat and less unhealthful saturated fat
- Eating more carbohydrates that have a low glycemic index (GI), which are carbohydrates that in general are less processed and higher in dietary fiber
- Not smoking
- Light or moderate alcohol use (which is associated with a lower risk of diabetes)
- Having a body mass index (BMI) under 25
- Having a smaller waist-to-hip ratio—which means having a waist measurement less than 34.6 inches for women and 36 inches for men

This may sound like a tall order, but the people in the study didn't need to adopt all of these habits at once to lower their risk. Overall, each lifestyle

Mind-Set Intervention: Avoid Defeatist Thinking

When you look at the list of low-risk, healthy diet and lifestyle habits, two things may come to mind: (1) These are the same habits you hear about all the time as helping you to lower your risk of a lot of health problems. (2) Many people have many high-risk factors, and making changes to adopt some healthier habits is hard. Both these thoughts are legitimate and true. There is a tremendous amount of over-lap between the things you can do to lower your risk of diabetes and numerous other health problems. If we treat our body the way it was evolutionarily designed to be treated, our weight is more likely to hover in a healthy range, our circulatory system will be less inflamed (and therefore less likely to form cholesterol blockages), our blood pressure will be lower, and our brain will have better circulation access to the health-promoting nutrients it needs to stay fit well into old age.

But we don't live in the world of our cave-dwelling ancestors. Jobs have moved largely out of the fields and into factories and office cubicles, and women have en-tered the workforce in huge numbers, leaving fewer people home during the day to plan and prepare meals. The overly invasive convenience food industry has stepped in to fill the void with foods that are quick, cheap, and crammed with calories, fat, and processed sugars. Technology has taken over all but a few lifestyle functions that used to burn a lot more calories. But there is a bright side: studies show that as little as 5 to 10 percent weight loss may help reverse your course toward diabe-tes, even if in the end you are still technically "overweight." The first step is to know where you stand on the blood glucose spectrum. And there's only one way to find that out: get tested.

factor in the low-risk category that an individual had was associated with a 35 percent lower risk of diabetes. Those who were in a low-risk category for only physical activity and diet (almost one in four of the participants) were 46 percent less likely to develop diabetes. Adding not smoking and moderate alcohol use to the healthy exercise and dietary habits (unfortunately, only about 6 percent of participants) resulted in an 82 percent lower risk of diabetes. Adding in not being overweight or not having a large waist circumference delivered an 89 percent lower risk of becoming diabetic.[44]

What's the bottom line? Eight in ten cases of diabetes in the older adults in this study were attributed to the *lack* of these four lifestyle habits: being moderately physically active; eating a diet higher in plant foods and lower in sugars, processed foods, and saturated fats; not smoking; and using alcohol in moderation (defined as no more than one drink per day for women and two drinks per day for men). This is without even factoring in being overweight or having a lot of belly fat! It stands to follow that if a lack of these healthy lifestyle factors is causing diabetes, then adopting these habits might help prevent eight in ten new cases of diabetes!

Diagnosing Prediabetes: The Testing Process

According to the American Diabetes Association (ADA), there are certain groups of people who should be tested and subsequently screened for prediabetes on a regular basis. Without obesity, screening should begin at age forty-five. Regardless of age, testing should be considered in all adults who are overweight (with a BMI of 25 or greater) and have additional risk factors, including:

- Physical inactivity
- First-degree relatives with diabetes
- High-risk race or ethnicity (African American, Latino, Native American, Asian American, Pacific Islander)
- Hypertension (greater than 140/90 mmHg or on medication for hypertension)
- HDL cholesterol level of less than 35 mg/dl and/or triglyceride level of greater than 250 mg/dl
- Women with polycystic ovary syndrome
- History of cardiovascular disease

According to the ADA, there are currently three different ways to be tested for prediabetes: a hemoglobin A1C test (also sometimes called a glycosylated hemoglobin test), a fasting plasma glucose test (FPG), and an oral glucose tolerance test (OGTT). Your blood glucose levels measured after these tests determine whether you have normal glucose metabolism, prediabetes, or diabetes. If you've had these tests done in the past, comparing results can give you hindsight. A fasting glucose test can sometimes be called something slightly different on a lab report (for example, it may also be called a "serum glucose" that then says "status: fasting" or something like that). If you're not sure what you're looking for, ask your health care provider.[45] All three of these blood tests should be conducted in a healthcare setting: your doctor may want to repeat the test on a second day to confirm a diagnosis. Urine tests are not useful for screening as they would only tell if you had poorly controlled blood glucose levels (because you were already diabetic). Let's take a closer look at each test.

Hemoglobin A1C Test

Sugar is "sticky," and when it's floating around in your blood, a certain amount of it will stick to the A1C component of your hemoglobin, which is a protein in your red blood cells. Having some glucose stuck to your hemoglobin is normal and is dictated by how much glucose is circulating in your blood. The amount of glucose adhered to these cells is expressed as a percentage, with 5.6 percent or less of the surface area of the A1C cell being covered with glucose considered normal. Hemoglobin cells live for approximately three months, so the hemoglobin A1C test result is considered a reflection of your average blood glucose levels over the previous two to three months. Because hemoglobin A1C doesn't change on a day-to-day basis, you don't need to be fasting for this test. A level of 5.7 percent to 6.4 percent is considered prediabetes. A hemoglobin A1C greater than or equal to 6.5 percent is considered diabetes.

Fasting Plasma Glucose (FPG) Test

This test requires you to fast overnight for at least eight to ten hours. Blood is drawn early the next day before you eat or drink anything. This is a test of how efficiently you're able to clear glucose out of your blood after several hours of overnight fasting. To interpret the test results, a normal fasting plasma glucose is less than 100 milligrams per deciliter (mg/dl). A fasting plasma glucose of 100 to 125 mg/dl is considered prediabetes. A fasting plasma glucose level at or above 126 mg/dl is considered diabetes.

Oral Glucose Tolerance Test (OGTT)

This test is used less often and requires an overnight fast. Your blood glucose is checked in the morning after fasting, after which you drink a concentrated glucose solution that contains 75 grams of glucose (the equivalent of drinking 23 ounces of soda very quickly). Your blood glucose is then checked again two hours later. This is a test of how well your body is able to respond to a large dose of glucose after an overnight fast. For some people, drinking the super-sweet glucose drink can be quite challenging! To interpret the OGTT results, a normal blood glucose is 140 mg/dl two hours after the glucose drink. A result of 140 to 199 mg/dl two hours after the drink is considered prediabetes. Equal to or greater than 200 mg/dl is considered diabetes.

It is also possible that a physician may diagnose diabetes based on a random plasma glucose of equal to or greater than 200 mg/dl in a patient with classic symptoms of hyperglycemia (such as increased thirst and frequent urination).

The testing for prediabetes is simple and noninvasive, and can be rolled into a routine physical. Now that you have a better understanding of what prediabetes is and how to be tested for it, it's time to move on to what's going in your body when you have prediabetes and how your diet and lifestyle affects the condition in either a positive or negative way. Managing prediabetes requires you to understand insulin resistance, and the next chapter provides a science lesson on that topic. Don't worry if physiology wasn't your favorite subject in school. You only need to understand enough to be able to visualize how what you eat, and whether you exercise or not, affects what's going on in your blood and subsequently with your health.

2

Insulin Resistance Explained

The key to reversing prediabetes is to truly understand what's going on in your body and how what you do affects it. My goal is to help you do that as naturally as possible so that you're only relying on medications to fill the gap between the progress you make with a healthy diet and activity and your goal. Many people with prediabetes don't even know they have the condition, and if they do, they understand very little about what that means. People are generally more familiar with diabetes, usually because of the experiences of friends or relatives who have the disease and are suffering its consequences. If you know you have prediabetes and have read up on it with the best intentions to make positive lifestyle changes, you may be having trouble figuring out just how to do it. Many people struggle with getting started. What should they be paying attention to? Is it the number of carbs on the food labels? Or sugars? Or calories? Is it okay to lose weight by any means necessary? How much exercise is enough to make it worth doing?

If you're overweight or obese, anything that will help you lose weight (as long as your overall nutritional needs are being met) is going to help reverse your prediabetes. Fine-tuning your diet to target the underlying insulin resistance can help with the weight-loss process in surprising ways. Insulin resistance can condition the body to have blood glucose fluctuations that affect food cravings and your energy level, as well as how you feel both physically and emotionally. If starting to adopt more healthy diet and exercise habits can make it so you're not moody and craving carbs and sugars all the time, you may start to believe that change is possible! Let's dive in and try to simplify the science.

Although a full consensus has yet to be reached as to why insulin resistance is so common today, evolutionarily speaking, this ability may have helped us store energy (as body fat) and preserve muscle (which helped preserve strength for hunting).[1] What once may have been meant to offer a shorter-term survival advantage, under the current conditions of our longer life spans, increased obesity, and sedentary lifestyle, is now contributing to a host of modern-day health problems. But what exactly is going on in the bloodstream, muscles, brain, and body fat, among other places, when you have insulin resistance? What can you do to normalize it?

The Hormone Insulin

Insulin is a hormone produced in the beta cells of the pancreas. Like other hormones in the body, insulin is released into the blood to travel around the body, exerting its effect. Insulin's major action is to dictate how the body utilizes energy. Glucose is the body's main energy source, and its presence in the blood stimulates insulin's release into circulation. Insulin secretion is critical to maintaining a stable and steady supply of glucose to the cells. According to the American Diabetes Association, the fasting blood glucose level should be below 100mg/dl. The normal range for a blood glucose level if you have not previously fasted for eight to ten hours depends on the time of day the blood was drawn. For nonpregnant adults, the normal range for a nonfasting blood glucose taken one to two hours after a meal is less than 180 milligrams per deciliter (mg/dl). A normal blood glucose taken before a meal is 70 to 130 mg/dl.[2]

If blood glucose levels drop too low, this condition is called hypoglycemia. If someone is hypoglycemic, they may start to feel a little fuzzy (like they're not thinking as clearly as usual), moody, and hungry—often for the carbohydrates the body uses to replenish its blood glucose supply (some people with insulin resistance report feeling intense cravings for carbs or sugar). If hypoglycemia progresses to dangerously low levels, which is only likely to happen to a diabetic who has taken too much injected insulin, unconsciousness can result—possibly even death. In hyperglycemia, when the blood glucose level is high, the body tries to produce as much insulin as it can in an effort to lower blood glucose levels. Over time this can be harder to accomplish if someone is insulin resistant and may eventually result in diabetes. The body knows that having excess glucose circulating around isn't good and will attempt to rid itself of the glucose by urinating it out through the kidneys. This accounts for the frequent urination and subsequent thirst seen as a symptom of diabetes.

At times when energy in the form of food exceeds what the body needs, insulin will promote the storage of glucose into the liver and muscle as glycogen, which are basically little "sugar cubes" of glucose stored as fuel for later use. When these reserves are filled, additional excess glucose is redirected to be stored as body fat—that important calorie reserve that was critical to human survival when food supplies were much more variable and often inadequate. Insulin promotes the storage of glucose as fat and glycogen and interferes with the breakdown of body fat (known as lipolysis). During conditions of drought or famine, it was good if insulin worked hard to encourage the storage of calorie reserves as body fat and make sure any withdrawn calories were being put to good use before letting them go. But this once-protective mechanism is backfiring today, making it tough to shed excess body fat that can become a health liability.

Because too much circulating insulin can make it hard to mobilize that dreaded belly fat, learning how to decrease insulin resistance is one of the most effective strategies for trimming your waistline. Like many hormones, the critical role insulin plays as an energy regulator is just one of its many jobs in the body. Insulin has many "target tissues" or cells throughout the body that rely on it for many important functions. The liver, muscles, blood vessels, pituitary gland, and brain all interact with insulin to perform different chemical activities in the body.

The Complex Actions of Insulin

What follows is a very basic description of the very complex actions of insulin in the body. To facilitate the clearance of sugar out of the blood and into the cells, where it can be used for fuel, insulin acts like a key connecting with a special lock on the cells, known as an insulin receptor. Every cell has anywhere from hundreds to thousands of insulin receptors. Once the insulin locates an insulin receptor on the cell, the insulin will connect and unlock the cell, allowing glucose to travel out of the blood and into the cell to be used as fuel. This process is very complex and involves a series of events geared toward allowing the cell access to an energy source.

Under normal circumstances the insulin receptors are sufficiently sensitive to the action of insulin to allow a cell to be opened using normal amounts of insulin. But some people don't use insulin as effectively as they should—they are *insulin resistant*—which makes their cells less sensitive to the action of insulin. The insulin comes knocking on the cell door, but the cell is holding the door shut and won't let the insulin do its job. The pancreas will sense this is happening and respond to this resistance by secreting more insulin into the blood—the goal being to overwhelm the cell with enough additional insulin that it will force the glucose into the cell. The result is that glucose clears out of the blood and into the cell, but at the expense of making the pancreas work harder than it should have to. If this goes untreated by diet, exercise, and weight loss (if needed), over time insulin resistance can exhaust the pancreas, rendering it less able to produce insulin. This is no different than what would happen if you put your car up on blocks, turned on the engine, and walked away: the engine would eventually burn out. When the pancreas no longer has the reserves to secrete extra insulin in response to insulin resistance, glucose will stop fully clearing out of the blood, which initially shows up as prediabetes.[5]

You can't rebuild the pancreas's ability to produce insulin once it's petered out; you can only learn how to work with it as a lifelong limitation. This means that once you have diabetes, you cannot cure it—the condition can only be managed. But with prediabetes you still have more insulin-producing ability than you would have if you let it go until you were diabetic, so the condition can potentially be reversed. It's much easier to prevent diabetes from happening than to take care of it once it occurs. Once excess insulin is secreted into the blood, it stands to negatively affect the many other functions of the body that are also influenced by insulin. In insulin resistance, it's muscle, fat, and liver cells that don't respond properly to insulin (mostly muscle cells, which gobble up 30 percent of the calories we eat).[4] But some cells remain sensitive to insulin, such as the ovaries, which react to being deluged with insulin due to insulin resistance triggered by other tissues. Insulin is a hormone, and this overexposure can cause imbalances in reproductive hormones, leading to the fertility problems seen in women with PCOS.

Genetic Predisposition and Incidence of Insulin Resistance

As mentioned earlier, it is believed that insulin resistance is a strongly inherited trait. If others in your family have prediabetes, diabetes, metabolic syndrome, or PCOS, your chances of having it too are increased. But inheriting insulin resistance is hardly black or white. There is great variability in how sensitively any one person processes insulin, much of which would fall within the normal range. *Not everyone with prediabetes goes on to develop diabetes, but the risk of doing so is high.* Muscle cells need a lot of glucose to sustain activity, which was particularly important when we expended a lot of energy hunting and gathering. But the central nervous system needs glucose too, to the tune of about 400 to 600 glucose calories a day to fuel the brain, spinal column, and nervous system.[5] If under conditions of physiological stress the muscle's cells gobbled up most of the incoming glucose in the form of dietary carbohydrates, the nervous system wouldn't get its fair share. Making the muscle cells somewhat resistant to insulin during these stressful times would help preserve some glucose in the blood for the brain and other nervous system tissues.

But what once may have been an important trait is not so helpful in a world where more people are overweight than not and life is sedentary. These risk factors have largely converted insulin resistance from a short-term survival strategy into a chronic condition. The bottom line is that insulin resistance has a long genetic history in humans and is strongly affected by diet, weight, activity, and lifestyle. If you have a genetic predisposition to it, the condition has a much greater chance of expressing itself if you're overweight and sedentary. There are many people with insulin resistance, prediabetes, and diabetes who would not have these conditions if they were active and at a healthy weight. At the same time, there are many healthy-weight, active people who would be insulin resistant, and possibly diabetic, if they were overweight and sedentary.

It's hard to say exactly how many people in the United States have insulin resistance because the condition is frequently undiagnosed until it turns into prediabetes or diabetes. In chapter 1 we discussed how common prediabetes and diabetes are—79 million people with prediabetes and 25.8 million people with diabetes—so you can imagine how many are already experiencing insulin resistance that has not yet progressed to prediabetes. These numbers have steadily increased over the past few decades and will continue to do so if we don't change the course of things. Determining just how insulin resistant someone might be, without having yet progressed to prediabetes, is not a perfect science. According to one study looking at insulin sensitivity in healthy individuals by insulin resistance expert Dr. Gerald Reaven, there was 600 percent variability in how sensitively study subjects utilized insulin, ranging from the most insulin sensitive to the least. Reaven estimates that about 25 percent of that variability is probably due to being overweight, 25 percent related to fitness level, and the remaining 50 percent possibly genetic.[6]

These findings suggest there is potentially a lot of room for positively influencing any genetic predisposition to diabetes with diet and lifestyle change. But research tells us that progression to diabetes among those with prediabetes is *not* inevitable. Studies have shown that people with prediabetes who lose at least 7 percent of their body weight (and keep as much of this weight off as possible!) and engage in moderate physical activity at least 150 minutes per week can prevent or delay diabetes—and in some people even return their blood glucose levels to normal. For a 250-pound man, this means maintaining a weight loss of 17.5 pounds; for a 200-pound woman, this means 14 pounds. And the exercise recommended is just half an hour, five days a week. Sounds possible, right? Without question, intensive lifestyle interventions are the most effective way to prevent or delay type 2 diabetes.[7]

Beyond the blood tests that diagnose prediabetes, insulin resistance doesn't have universal signs and symptoms. But in my experience, many people with insulin resistance have similar complaints. These include the following:

- Fluctuations in energy level throughout the day—some start off energetic but crash in the afternoon
- Frequent hunger and, after eating, not feeling full for long
- Binge eating at meals
- Constant cravings for sweets and other refined carbohydrates, like white bread, crackers, or pasta
- Irritability and feeling shaky if they go too long without eating (this is the central nervous system acting up), which might not be long at all compared to people without insulin resistance
- Severe intolerance to very low-calorie diets, particularly those that severely limit carbohydrates

Of course these signs and symptoms can occur and be unrelated to insulin resistance, but in my practice these are commonly expressed complaints. What's striking about some people with insulin resistance is a feeling that food has an unusual hold over them that they don't think other people experience. They often describe a feeling of being "addicted" to refined carbohydrates and sweets.

Improving Insulin Resistance Through Diet and Exercise

The simplest way to start visualizing how we should be eating and changing our lifestyle is to imagine that primitive caveperson. We're not going back to being hunters and gatherers, but let's look at how life was different then: the primary difference being the level of activity. Compared to the modern-day coach potato or cubicle dweller, hunters and gatherers burned hundreds, if not thousands, more calories daily. Acquiring and preparing food required a lot more effort physically, and once eaten, the food itself demanded more effort from the digestive tract. Food was much more fibrous and needed a lot more chewing in the mouth and grinding up in the stomach to get it down to a liquid form for absorption. The act

Mind-Set Intervention: Don't Let the Science Scare You

For many people it makes a big difference to finally get what's going on in their body with all this blood sugar stuff. It's one thing to be told to "just lose weight" or "cut back on your carbohydrates" and another thing to really understand why these strategies can make a real difference. But it's also easy to feel like you're drowning in the scientific details if you have prediabetes. Focus on what you can do about it. Try to keep an open mind and have no rigid timelines within which you feel you have to accomplish things. It probably took years to get where you are, so your reality isn't going to change overnight.

Take baby steps when implementing healthy changes in your diet and lifestyle. When you first start making changes, you may notice some improvements fairly quickly in your weight and how you feel—a little lighter on your feet, a little more energetic, maybe a little more mood-stable. What matters most is that you hang in there for the long haul, even when the road gets bumpy. This is about the rest of your life, not just a few months. You want the changes you make to be sustainable. Keep telling yourself, you can do this! Put sticky notes on your kitchen cabinets, on the dashboard of your car, or on your computer at work as reminders that it is possible. Now is the time to take action!

of eating was more rigorous for the body and dragged out the eating and digestion processes. Compare that to the effort needed to chug down a sugar-loaded soda!

It is therefore genetically and physiologically more "normal" for us to eat food that is as minimally processed as possible. We should also deliberately seek out every available opportunity to physically move the body throughout the day. Although some people develop diabetes without being overweight and sedentary, for most of them, the writing has been on the wall for some time that diabetes is in their future. Fortunately, new research supports the idea that making even very modest changes in diet and lifestyle may be enough to help postpone or even sideline the disease. Several studies have shown that diet and lifestyle interventions can prevent or delay progression to diabetes, two of the most widely noted being the Finnish Diabetes Prevention Study and the Diabetes Prevention Program. Both looked at diabetes prevention and cardiovascular disease prevention, as these two diseases are so closely linked. Let's discuss the compelling findings of these two studies.

The Finnish Diabetes Prevention Study

The first major research study on lifestyle and diabetes prevention came out of Finland in 2001. In the Finnish Diabetes Prevention Study, researchers randomly assigned 522 middle-aged, overweight subjects (172 men, 350 women, mean age of fifty-five, mean BMI of 31) with impaired glucose tolerance to either an intervention or control group.[8] The people in the control group were given some oral information about diet and exercise, along with a two-page pamphlet to take home at the start of the study and again at annual visits, but no specific programs were offered to them. This could be compared to what many people traditionally get in the doctor's office who do not then move on to more ongoing, individualized counseling with a registered dietitian.

In contrast, those in the intervention group received individual nutrition counseling aimed at reducing weight and total intake of fat and saturated fat and increasing intake of dietary fiber and physical activity (which was specifically tailored to them based on three-day food records they filled out four times a year). The goals of the intervention were for the participants to lose at least 5 percent of their starting body weight, to reduce fat intake to 30 percent of their total calories and saturated fat to less than 10 percent of total calories, and to increase fiber intake to at least 15 grams per 1,000 calories consumed. Fruits, vegetables, whole grains, low-fat dairy, lean meats, tub margarine spreads, and heart-healthy monounsaturated fats were encouraged. Participants in this group also received individualized advice on both aerobic and strength activities, with an overall activity goal of exercising at a moderate pace for at least thirty minutes a day. The average follow-up for the study was 3.2 years per participant.

The results were quite interesting. During the course of the study, the incidence of diabetes was 58 percent lower in the intervention group than in the control group, even though a large portion of the subjects didn't meet their weight-loss or diet goals. Some findings:

- Of the 522 participants, 86 were diagnosed with diabetes during the study—27 in the intervention group and 59 in the control group.
- The likelihood of developing diabetes was directly related to how many lifestyle goals were met—those who made significant changes experienced the greatest reduction in risk, whereas those who didn't make any changes had a 35 percent chance of becoming diabetic during the three years of the study, which is generally what would be expected in these high-risk patients.
- The average amount of weight lost wasn't much, but the odds of becoming diabetic were substantially lower in those who lost the target 5 percent. For someone who started out weighing 220 pounds, for example, this meant losing only about 11 pounds.
- Even in the subjects who didn't lose any weight, hitting a relatively conservative target of more than four hours of exercise a week was tied to a significantly lower likelihood of developing diabetes.
- The researchers feel it is likely that any kind of activity—whether sports, gardening, household tasks, or work-related activity—was similarly beneficial for preventing diabetes.

The study subjects in the intervention group had a lot of support— seven sessions with a nutritionist during the first year and once every three months thereafter. But they also had a relatively low dropout rate, which the researchers suggest makes the case that people with prediabetes are motivated to avoid diabetes and that pessimism about overweight, sedentary people's ability to make change is unwarranted.

The Diabetes Prevention Program (DPP)

The other much larger study published in 2002, the Diabetes Prevention Program, confirmed that intensive lifestyle change is the most potent way to avoid diabetes, even when stacked up against diabetes-prevention medication.[9] In this study 3,234 nondiabetic participants (average age of fifty-one, mean BMI of 34) were recruited through twenty-seven clinical centers around the United States. Forty-five percent of the participants were from minority groups at higher risk of developing diabetes, including African Americans, Native Alaskans, American Indians, Asian Americans, Hispanics/Latinos, and Pacific Islanders. Study participants were randomly divided into three different groups:

1. Standard lifestyle recommendations plus the diabetes drug metformin (also known as Glucophage) at a dose of 850 milligrams twice daily.
2. Standard lifestyle recommendations plus a placebo, or dummy pill, twice daily.
3. Lifestyle intervention group that received intensive training in diet, physical activity, and behavior modification.

The standard lifestyle recommendations for the medication and placebo groups were provided as written information, plus an annual twenty- to thirty-minute individual session that emphasized the importance of a healthy lifestyle. Participants were encouraged to lose weight and increase their physical activity—sound like your last doctor's appointment? The goals of the intensive lifestyle intervention group were to lose at least 7 percent of their body weight through a healthy, low-calorie, low-fat diet and to exercise at a moderate intensity for at least 150 minutes a week (or about thirty minutes five days a week). The participants were individually educated on how to achieve these goals using a sixteen-lesson curriculum covering diet, exercise, and behavior modification during the first twenty-four weeks of the study. The curriculum was designed to be flexible, individualized, and culturally sensitive. Subsequent monthly individual or group sessions reinforced the information. The average follow-up was 2.8 years per participant.

The results of the DPP study were surprising. The incidence of diabetes was 58 percent lower in the lifestyle intervention group (same as the Finnish study) and 31 percent lower in the metformin group compared to the placebo group. Almost twice as many people in the lifestyle intervention group avoided developing type 2 diabetes during the time of the study than those who got standard education and took diabetes medication. Some interesting findings:

- Over the three-year period, it was estimated that 28.9 percent of the placebo group and 21.7 percent of the metformin group developed diabetes, compared with only 14.4 percent of the intensive lifestyle intervention group.

- The lifestyle intervention was highly effective in all groups regardless of sex, race, ethnicity, or age, supporting its usefulness in all age, ethnic, and cultural groups. Researchers believe that weight loss—achieved through better eating habits and exercise—reduced the risk of diabetes by improving the ability of the body to use insulin and process glucose.

- Lifestyle changes worked particularly well for people age sixty and older, reducing their risk of developing diabetes by 71 percent.

Long-Term Benefits:
The Diabetes Prevention Program Outcomes Study

For intervention studies like the DPP, the hope is that the intervention put in play during the research phase provides lasting benefits for its participants. To see if that was the case, a follow-up study, the DPP Outcomes Study (DPPOS), followed the participants over the five years after the intervention.[10] Had the gains participants made during the trial been maintained after the study ended? By the end of five years, researchers found that those with prediabetes who had their blood sugar return to normal during the DPP, even if it was only for a short period of time, were 56 percent less likely to develop type 2 diabetes in the five years after the study compared with those who remained persistently prediabetic. And it didn't even seem to matter how the lower blood sugar was achieved—whether through diet changes only, weight loss only, increased exercise, or a combination of these lifestyle changes. An additional follow-up study of the DPPOS after ten years found the lifestyle group's chance of developing diabetes was still reduced by 34 percent.[11]

Besides diabetes prevention, another major goal of the DPP was to see if cardiovascular risk factors could be positively affected by the changes designed to prevent diabetes. A ten-year follow-up study of the DPPOS, released in 2013, looked at whether there were long-term differences in cardiovascular risk factors and use of cholesterol and blood pressure–lowering medications in the DPP intervention group compared with the other groups (those on metformin or a placebo).[12] Major reductions were seen for blood pressure and unhealthy LDL cholesterol and triglyceride levels, along with significant increases in healthy HDL cholesterol levels, in all three groups. When it came to medications, however, cholesterol and blood pressure medication use was lower in the lifestyle intervention group.

What can we conclude from these findings? Lifestyle intervention helped the study subjects achieve similar long-term improvements in their cardiovascular risk factors as the other groups, with less need to rely on medications. Given that cholesterol-lowering medications can have significant side effects (and they're not designed to be an alternative to diet and exercise anyway), it's nice to know the same diet and lifestyle strategies seem to be able to kill two birds with one stone.

The Importance of Scientific Studies

Research has repeatedly demonstrated that *diabetes is a preventable disease*. In a perfect world, up to 89 percent of type 2 diabetes could be avoided by paying more attention to how we eat and getting some regular exercise. And exercise doesn't need to be any more aggressive than taking a walk. The sooner you get on the prevention bandwagon, the better. If you're overweight and sedentary, or have family members with diabetes, regardless of whether you have other risk factors, diabetes may be in your future. You should take steps now to reduce your risk. If you do have additional risk factors—like PCOS or metabolic syndrome, or you've already had an elevated blood glucose screening—it's definitely time to pay attention and shift into gear with an action plan. Remember, diabetes can't be cured, but you may be able to prevent or delay its onset by getting serious about diet, exercise, and behavioral strategies that will improve your physical and emotional health as well as your quality of life. The information presented in part 2 of this book will help you get there.

Part 2

THE PREDIABETES DIET PLAN: PREVENTING DIABETES

3

Managing Your Carbohydrate Intake to Reverse Prediabetes

Now that you have a better understanding of prediabetes and its causes—and why you should eat differently and exercise more to manage the condition—let's talk specifics about how to make that happen. While weight loss is the most potent way to try to reverse prediabetes if you're overweight, in this chapter, we'll look at how what you eat affects your insulin response.

Your Diet and Insulin Resistance

What you eat affects your insulin response, and these effects will differ whether someone is insulin resistant or not. As we covered in chapter 2, insulin resistance is a complex condition associated with many different health problems, including diabetes, gestational diabetes, metabolic syndrome, polycystic ovary syndrome (PCOS), cardiovascular disease, and several different types of cancer. But there's good news: controlling insulin resistance lowers the risks of all these conditions. Before reviewing what happens during "normal" insulin and blood sugar (glucose) metabolism (the terms "blood sugar" and "glucose" are used interchangeably throughout this book), here are some facts:

- Glucose is the body's primary source of fuel, feeding all of the body's cells, including muscles and organs (such as the liver and the brain) as well as body fat.

- There has to be some sugar in the blood at all times as it's the fuel of the human body. A normal (nonfasting) blood sugar generally runs somewhere between 70 and 115 milligrams per deciliter (mg/dl).
- The glucose that's in our bloodstream is a combination of glucose released from glucose reserves in the liver, called glycogen, and glucose released into the blood after the digestion of food, mainly from dietary carbohydrates.
- When you eat carbohydrates, it takes about sixty to ninety minutes for the majority of the carbs to be digested down to their most basic units (glucose) and released into your bloodstream.
- How rapidly those sugars arrive in your bloodstream depends on how easy the carbs you just ate are to digest. In general, refining or processing a carbohydrate before it's consumed is, in a way, like predigesting it: your body is going to have less work to do on the inside to finish up the digestion process and release the sugars into the blood. For example, soda is already "liquid sugar," so it will be released into your blood as glucose faster than the sugars from a bowl of plain oatmeal, which is eaten in a much more natural form.
- The rate of carbohydrate digestion—and therefore the rate at which your blood glucose levels will rise after eating a carb—can be influenced by the glycemic index (GI) or glycemic load (GL) of a food. These terms are discussed in greater detail later in the book.
- How much sugar will ultimately be released into your bloodstream is directly proportional to how much carbohydrate you ate or drank—that is, a large portion of carbs will result in a greater rise in blood glucose than a smaller portion.

Now that we've reviewed the basics of blood sugar, let's look at blood sugar processing. What happens during "normal" insulin and blood sugar metabolism, and how are things different if you're insulin resistant? Let's break the process down into steps with Joan, our imaginary non-insulin-resistant woman:

1. Joan hasn't eaten in a while, so she has a normal, baseline amount of sugar circulating in her bloodstream.

2. For lunch, Joan eats a turkey sandwich and an orange, along with a glass of milk. The bread from the sandwich, the milk, and the orange all contain carbs.

3. Within about an hour of eating, the majority of the carbs Joan ate for lunch have showed up as glucose in her blood. She now has her baseline blood sugars plus the sugars from the carbs she ate for lunch.

4. The excess sugars from the foods Joan just digested don't want to linger in her bloodstream for long. They want to move out and enter her cells all around her body so the cells can be energized and her blood sugar can return to normal.

5. For the sugar to enter the cells, the cells need to be unlocked with the help of insulin, which is released by the pancreas, an organ that sits behind the stomach, close to where the sugars exit the intestine and enter the bloodstream. (Besides being involved in sugar metabolism, the pancreas also secretes digestive enzymes into the intestine to help break down food into nutrients.) Shortly after the glucose arrives in the bloodstream, it circulates through the pancreas, which measures the blood glucose and releases enough insulin into the blood to clear the excess glucose from the blood.

6. Now Joan has insulin circulating in her bloodstream, along with glucose. Think of insulin as a bunch of little keys that rush around the body, unlocking the cells so glucose can exit the bloodstream and enter the cells to be incinerated for energy.

7. In order for the insulin keys to unlock the cells, they must first connect with "key holes" on the cells called insulin receptors. Once the insulin and insulin receptors connect, the cells open up and allow the sugar to enter.

This whole process takes about two hours, at which point Joan's blood sugar should be back within a normal range. But how is this different for someone who has insulin resistance? Let's take a look at James, our imaginary man with insulin resistance:

1. James just had lunch with Joan and ate the same thing (a turkey sandwich, an orange, and a glass of milk).

2. Like Joan, James's pancreas got the message about sugar in the blood and released what it thought should be the amount of insulin

needed to unlock the cells and clear the excess sugars out of the blood. In his case, however, the insulin has trouble unlocking the cells.

3. When the insulin from James's pancreas approaches the cells to hook up with the insulin receptors, the insulin and the receptors don't connect as efficiently as they should. It's like having a key that looks like the right key to a door, but when you put it in the lock, it won't turn to unlock, so the door remains locked. On a cellular level, the receptor is resisting the action of the insulin, hence the term insulin resistance. The pancreas senses that this is happening—the sugars just aren't clearing out of the bloodstream as efficiently as they should—and it responds by secreting more insulin into the blood. The idea is to overwhelm the cells with extra insulin, forcing them to accept the glucose. In the early stages, the pancreas has plenty of reserve insulin-making ability, so the sugars do eventually clear out of the blood. The problem is that over time this extra work can exhaust the pancreas to the point where it's no longer able to secrete enough extra insulin to overcome insulin resistance.

Over time, this process can eventually lead to diabetes in anyone with insulin resistance. The pancreas may eventually wear out from overuse. When glucose from carbs comes calling for insulin to help escort it out of the blood, the pancreas no longer has the ability to produce enough insulin. The result is prediabetes and maybe eventually diabetes.

The Prediabetes-Carbohydrate Connection

In recent years those trying to lose weight or "get healthy" have been at risk for jumping on the low-carb bandwagon. The problem with this approach is that it discounts a large body of research supporting the value of including unprocessed carbohydrates in one's diet for prevention of heart disease, diabetes, and cancer. Low-carb diets have not been proven to result in lasting weight loss. But that doesn't mean there isn't room for improvement in the way the average American consumes carbs. The reality is that most of us eat far too many calories, considering our ever-dwindling levels of physical activity. According to the most recent 2009–2010 National Health and Nutrition Examination Survey (NHANES) conducted by the CDC's National Center for Health Statistics, which describes trends in our daily food intake over the past three decades, American women increased their daily calorie consumption between 1971 and 2010 from 1,542 calories a day to 1,778 calories. During the same period the calorie intake for men increased from 2,450 calories a day to 2,512 calories.[1]

These differences may not sound like much, but an extra 236 calories a day for women adds up to an extra 86,140 calories a year—or potentially thirty-five pounds of weight gain. For men the extra 63 calories a day accrues to 22,630 extra calories a year—or about 6.5 pounds of weight gain. Women have accumulated excess calories at a rate of almost four times that of men! And none of this takes into account how much less active we are now on average when compared with activity levels in 1971.

Equally distressing, from 1970 to 2005 our intake of added sugars has increased a whopping 19 percent, which on its own increased the average American's calorie intake by 76 calories a day. According to food trend surveys from the US Department of Agriculture, the per-person amount of added sugars and sweeteners in the American diet totaled 142 pounds a year in 2005, up from 119 pounds a year in 1970. The most striking change between 1970 and 2005 is the availability of corn sweetener, which increased by 387 percent, driven mostly by high fructose corn sweetener (HFCS), the use of which increased in the food supply from 3 percent in the 1970s to a current 76 percent of all corn sweeteners.[2] The jury is still out as to whether there's anything uniquely unhealthy about HFCSs, but what isn't debatable is the damaging health effects of eating (or drinking) too much sugar.

Excessive sugar intake is contributing to a worldwide epidemic of obesity and heart disease, and is increasingly being tied to escalating rates of diabetes. According to the American Heart Association, in 2001 to 2004 the usual intake of added sugars for Americans was 22.2 teaspoons a day (333 calories' worth), which is more than triple the association's recommendation of no more than 6 teaspoons of added sugar for women (about 100 calories' worth) and 9 teaspoons for men (about 150 calories' worth).[3] Compare that to the average 17 teaspoons of sugar in a typical 20-ounce soda and it's easy to see how sugar intake in the United States has spun out of control. Fortunately, research published recently in the *American Journal of Clinical Nutrition* suggests we may be backing off on our sugar intake, mostly by cutting back on soda, but we still have a long way to go toward curbing our national sweet tooth.[4]

Chasing Dietary Fads

America has a history full of dietary fads and extremes, and the 1980s was the decade to demonize fat. Research at the time suggested that eating too much fat was raising people's risk of heart disease, so scientists and health advocates began clamoring for us to cut back on dietary fat. Initially these recommendations made sense. Too much unhealthy saturated and trans fat is tied to cardiovascular problems, and fatty foods are high in calories, with every gram eaten adding 9 calories as opposed to carbohydrates and proteins, which deliver only 4 calories per gram. After a few years it started to become clear that trying to avoid fat may take a bite out of blood cholesterol levels (studies began to show a decline in cholesterol levels from the early 1980s to 2002, although some of this was due in part to the increased use of cholesterol-lowering medications), but the fat-free part wasn't helping us with our ever-expanding waistlines. How could this be? What we now understand more is that most carbs don't contain much protein, which helps slow the passage of food from your stomach into your intestines, helping you feel fuller, longer. Also, many people were loading up on refined "white flour" carbs that digest quickly, causing a rapid rise in blood glucose and triggering a hefty demand for insulin—and subsequently more hunger. Many also forgot that "fat-free" doesn't mean "calorie-free." Refined carbs don't control hunger for long, which caused many people to continually graze on high-carb, low-protein foods throughout the day, leading to an actual increase in their calorie intake.

By the end of the fat-free trend, it was evident that simply trimming fat wasn't the answer. You also have to control calories if you want to lose weight. Furthermore, some fats are healthy for us—like the omega-3 fats found in fish, walnuts, and flaxseeds; monounsaturated fats such as olive and canola oil and those found in nuts, seeds, and avocados; and the polyunsaturated fats in seeds and vegetable oils. When used in moderation, these fats also slow down digestion, helping us feel more satisfied and allowing us to hold our hunger at bay for longer. The rich taste and creamy mouthfeel of these fats also enhances our enjoyment of eating, which may help many people feel less deprived. The bottom line is that it really comes down to the principle of the Two Qs: quality and quantity.

We could have saved our future selves from the low-carb fad of the 1990s and early 2000s by opting instead for whole grains, like whole grain bread, oatmeal, quinoa, and brown rice. It seems we're always looking for that perfect diet that is high in one thing and low in something else. But the best dietary approach is to focus on the middle ground. The prediabetes diet plan recommendation is to eat a diet moderate in less-processed carbs that are spread out in smaller doses over meals and snacks, and pair them with lean proteins and small amounts of healthful fats wherever possible to help each eating episode feel more filling.

Understanding Carbohydrates

When trying to figure out whether what you're eating contains carbs or not, the first question to ask is, does the food come from a plant? Fruits, vegetables (although starchy vegetables, which we'll discuss later, are the only significant sources), and grains all contain carbohydrates. Milk and yogurt also contain carbs in the form of lactose. Although cheese is made from milk, most of the carbohydrate is consumed by the healthy bacteria used to make the cheese, so cheese contains little to no carbohydrate. These are all what we call "good carbs," or carbohydrates that contribute a lot of healthy nutrients to the diet in addition to glucose for energy. Then there are the "empty calorie" carbs (so-called bad carbs) that have little to offer nutritionally beyond glucose calories—items like soda, candy, cakes, cookies, ice cream, chips, and other snack foods. These foods provide few vitamins and minerals, no fiber, often contain large amounts of unhealthy trans or saturated fats, and are the source of many excess calories.

Studies show that Americans consume too much added sugar and processed carbs and not enough healthful, unprocessed carbs that can do your body good. It's not that there is no room for special treats. Even the USDA's Choose My Plate recommendation allows for some "just for fun" calories once your other needs for healthful foods are met. The problem is that many Americans are filling up on processed sugars and refined carbs without getting enough of the good stuff first! If you go out of your way to include fruits and vegetables at meals and snacks—even if they're not your favorite foods, so not everything you're loading up on is calorie heavy—it's possible to make room for a small daily serving of something to indulge your sweet tooth.

Including Carbs in Your Diet

The "good carbs" are critical as a source of easy-to-access energy, so you shouldn't eliminate them completely. Carbs are quickly converted to glucose, which acts as a fuel source for every cell in the body. The key is to remember the Two Qs: Choose the best-quality carbs while watching the quantity. According to the 2010 Dietary Guidelines for Americans, the percentage of calories that should come from carbohydrates, proteins, and fats is not one size fits all. It depends on your preferences, overall health, and activity level. One thing's for sure, though: you can't live without carbs. What too often gets lost in the discussion about how much carbohydrate is healthy is the incredibly valuable role carbohydrates play in keeping us adequately nourished and feeling energetic—if you choose the right ones.

Foods that contain carbs make many valuable contributions to the body. As mentioned, the biggest consumers of glucose are our muscles and central nervous system (the brain, spinal cord, and nerves). Brain cells need twice as much energy as the other cells in the body. The central nervous system needs about 400 to 600 calories' worth of carbs a day for those tissues to be fully fueled, accounting for the sensations of weakness, moodiness, trouble focusing, and, in some people, actual shakiness when we go too long without eating. In many people these symptoms cause intense cravings for carbs because your body knows what will bring your blood glucose levels back into the range that's right for you. For those with a particularly sweet tooth, the call may be more specifically for something sugary. Why wouldn't the body feel this way? We have instincts just like animals, and if our blood glucose levels are drifting down because of carb deprivation, it makes perfect sense that the brain would stimulate you to seek them out. This also explains why some people simply cannot tolerate very low-carb diets, such as the Atkins nutritional approach. It physically makes them feel weak, cranky, and sick!

Starches (also known as complex carbohydrates). Carbohydrates are classified as either starches, sugars, or dietary fiber (fiber will be discussed later in this chapter). Starches are long chains of sugar units hooked together. Because starches are large molecules, when they hit your tongue they don't taste sweet. During digestion the sugar units are separated from one another by digestive enzymes and are ultimately released into the bloodstream in their most basic form, as simple sugars (glucose, galactose, and fructose), with glucose being the main form used for energy. Your best choices for starches are whole grains because they have not been processed to remove their dietary fiber and health-promoting phytonutrients (disease-fighting chemicals in plant foods that support immune function, squelch inflammation, and act as natural antioxidants). Refined carbs, on the other hand—like white rice, regular pasta, processed cereals, and other grains made with white flour—have been stripped of their fiber and phytonutrients. Although in the United States most refined carbs are fortified with some vitamins, iron, and other minerals, you can't add back the phytonutrients. They're gone forever.

Sugars. Unlike starches, sugars are either single-unit molecules (glucose, fructose, and galactose) that can be absorbed whole, or two units hooked together (sucrose, lactose, and maltose) that need to break down into single units for absorption. Some people lack enough of the enzyme lactase that breaks lactose down into glucose and galactose, causing symptoms of lactose intolerance (diarrhea, bloating, and gas). Sugars are small molecules so they can snuggle right into your taste buds and stimulate that sensation of "sweet." Sugars can be either naturally occurring in fruit and dairy foods (packaged along with other healthful nutrients) or added during processing (nutritionally devoid of anything but sugar calories).

Starchy vegetables. Most vegetables contain very little carbohydrate. They're mostly water and some fiber. For this reason they make a great "filler food" that we won't officially count as carb foods in our discussions about managing carb intake. There is a short list of starchy vegetables (their starch content makes them look more like bread than broccoli under a microscope) that we count as a starch choice at a meal. These include potatoes, sweet potatoes, yams, winter squash, corn, peas, beans, and plantains. You want to treat starchy vegetables as a starch when meal planning. Don't eliminate them from your diet, though. Brightly colored sweet potatoes and winter squash are far more nutrient-dense than white potatoes because of their high carotenoid content (a natural antioxidant phytonutrient), and they have a lower glycemic index (more on that later). French fries—sadly listed as the number-one consumed vegetable in the

United States!—should not be regularly counted as a starch. Rather, these should go on the "occasional treat list" because they are often fried in unhealthy fats and loaded with calories.

Recommendations from the Professionals

Choosing moderate amounts of whole grains, starchy vegetables, and beans to provide the bulk of your carbohydrate intake will add a lot of fiber and other healthful nutrients to your diet. Focusing on carbs across the board as "bad" and cutting them out of your diet entirely isn't a good idea. This will likely leave you feeling tired and deprived, robbing you of many nutrients your body needs for good health and optimal function. The official word on how we should be managing our carb intake comes from government agencies like the US Department of Agriculture, the Centers for Disease Control (CDC), the US Department of Health and Human Services (HHS), and the National Institutes of Health (NIH). The following recommendations were gleaned from the 2010 Dietary Guidelines for Americans:[5] The recommended dietary allowance (RDA) for carbohydrates, which should be viewed as the bare minimum for good health and energy, is 130 grams. An example of what 130 grams of carbs looks like is four servings of grains, two servings of fruits, two servings of dairy (milk or yogurt), and three servings nonstarchy vegetables (notice the healthy carb-controlled meal plan taking shape).

Also from the 2010 Dietary Guidelines for Americans: Sugars can be naturally present in foods (such as the fructose in fruit or the lactose in milk), or added sugars, like sugars and syrups added at the table or during processing or preparation (such as high fructose corn syrup in sweetened beverages and baked products). The "sugar" content listed on a food label includes both naturally occurring and added sugars. To see how much of this sugar is likely to be added, look at the ingredient list on the food label. The closer to the top that a form of sugar is listed, the higher the content of added sugars. Labels can be confusing. For example, consider 100 percent orange juice. Even though all the carbs in the OJ are naturally occurring fructose from the oranges, to the uneducated consumer it looks like OJ is loaded with "sugar"—however, the ingredient list will show only oranges and maybe water, no added sugars.

The body's response to sugars is basically the same whether they are naturally present or added to the food. Natural sugars from fruit (fructose) and dairy (lactose) have an advantage because they're packaged along with other healthful nutrients, whereas added sugars supply calories but few or no nutrients. Eating a lot of added sugars (from foods or beverages, including that sugar-loaded morning coffee) has been tied to weight gain and poor-quality diets. On a food label, any of the following terms indicate an added sugar:

Brown sugar	Lactose
Corn sweetener	Maltose
Corn syrup	Malt syrup
Dextrose	Maple syrup
Fructose	Molasses
Fruit juice concentrates	Raw sugar
Glucose	Sucrose
High fructose corn syrup	Sugar
Honey	Syrup
Invert sugar	White sugar

Here are some other helpful tips from the 2010 Dietary Guidelines:

- Aim for at least 2½ cups of vegetables per day to reduce your risk of many chronic diseases.
- The majority of our fruit servings should come from whole fruit. One serving a day of 100 percent fruit juice (1 cup) can add some important vitamins and minerals to the diet (but no fiber), but drinking too much juice can contribute unwanted weight gain. Dried fruit can be included as well, but only about 2 tablespoons give you the same amount of carbs and calories as a whole piece of fruit.
- Legumes—such as dry beans and peas—are especially rich in fiber and protein and should be consumed several times a week.
- Half or more of all your grains should come from whole grains, such as whole grain cereal, bread and crackers, brown rice, barley, quinoa, and whole wheat pasta. Nutrient-rich whole grains have been linked to lower rates of obesity, heart disease, and diabetes, and they are more filling than refined carbohydrates.

- The percentage of your daily calories that should come from carbs ranges from 45 to 65 percent, depending on your individual health needs (at the lower end in the case of those who are insulin resistant, higher than this for endurance athletes). Added sugars should be limited.

- Your daily dietary fiber intake (for both men and women) should be 14 grams per every 1,000 calories consumed, or on average between 20 and 35 grams of fiber a day. Dietary surveys suggest most Americans eat only about half that, or 14 grams a day. Ideally, most of that fiber would come from naturally occurring fibers in whole grains, fruits, and vegetables (as opposed to foods that have fibers added to them (such as yogurt or white bread with added fiber, which doesn't count as a whole grain).

There is ample reason to include some good-quality carbohydrate in your diet. Unless you drown them in butter or cheese sauce, quality carbs provide fiber, phytonutrients, and satisfaction with your meal without loading you down with excess calories. But it's worth repeating: it's all about the quantity. There are no free rides when it comes to carbs, or any other calorie-containing food for that matter. You can still gain weight by eating bran cereal, brown rice, or whole wheat pasta if you eat more than you need to balance your calorie intake and activity.

The Glycemic Index and Glycemic Load

During the low-carb diet craze, many people became familiar with the term "glycemic index" (GI). The glycemic index is a numerical system that measures the rate at which carbs from food arrive in the bloodstream as glucose in the hours after they are eaten. The original research was conducted in the mid-1980s and was designed to help people with diabetes determine how different foods might affect their blood sugar. To determine GI, a 50-gram portion of a carb-containing food is fed to non-diabetic volunteers, and their blood glucose levels are then checked at intervals over the following hours. All foods tested are compared to the response of a dose of pure oral glucose (this is what you drink for a glucose tolerance test), which has a rating of 100. The test food is rated based on the percentage it raises blood sugar compared to oral glucose (for example, unsweetened oatmeal raises blood sugar 55 percent as much as glucose, so the GI is 55).

A low GI food has a rating of 55 or less; a medium GI food is rated 56 to 69; and a high GI food is rated 70 or higher. Several factors affect GI, including how acidic the food is, how much the food is processed or cooked, whether it contains fiber, or if it is eaten along with other foods. In general, foods that raise blood glucose more rapidly will have a higher GI rating. However, portion size limits how much any food can raise blood sugar levels regardless of its GI. Some foods—like a big bagel or a cup of cooked white rice—can easily deliver a 50-gram dose of carbs. Other foods—like carrots, for example, which were routinely deemed "bad for you" during the low-carb days for having a high GI—are rarely eaten in 50-gram doses (that would be about 1½ pounds of carrots!) or alone without other foods. A limitation of the GI system is that solely focusing on the ratings of different foods may distract from the fact that portion control is still extremely important.

To account for usual portions of carb-containing foods, another system has been developed called the glycemic load (GL), which takes into account the GI and the amount of carbohydrate in a typical serving (within which carrots rate very favorably). A low GL is less than 10, moderate is 11 to 19, and high is 20 or above. The simple interpretation of

Facts About Fiber

Fiber is a type of carbohydrate that human beings can't digest. As such, we need to sift through dietary fiber during digestion to extract the digestible carbs from the food, which increases the time it takes for them to show up as glucose in our blood. Research shows that dietary fiber may help improve blood glucose levels in those with diabetes.[6] Dietary fiber also increases the feeling of fullness after a meal. Dietary fibers are categorized as water soluble and water insoluble. Water-soluble fibers can help lower dangerous LDL-cholesterol levels, and are found in oats, peas, beans, apples, citrus fruits, carrots, barley, and psyllium.[7] Water-insoluble fibers are strong contributors to digestive health because they add bulk to the stool, speeding up the passage of waste through your gut. Fruit and vegetables (particularly the skins), whole wheat and wheat bran products, nuts, and seeds are all good sources of insoluble fiber. Many plant foods contain both soluble and insoluble fibers. When a grain is stripped of its fiber, it's also stripped of the "germ," which is where most of the vitamins, minerals, and phytonutrients are stored.

GI/GL is that the closer the food is to the form it occurs in nature, the lower the GI/GL, and the more processed it is, the higher the GI/GL.

Pairing carbs with proteins and healthy fats (keeping portion control in mind) also tempers the effect on blood sugar of any carbohydrate. The glycemic index can be a useful system to use alongside a carb-controlled diet as a means of increasing your intake of foods that are healthier and more filling. But again, using the GI or GL systems alone to determine what you should be eating is too simplistic because it doesn't account for the amount of carbs or calories in a food. Just because a food has a low GI does not mean you can eat all you want. For more on the glycemic index and glycemic load of foods, visit www.glycemicindex.com.

The Skinny on Artificial Sweeteners

As concern about excessive carb intake has increased, an ever-expanding list of artificial sweeteners has infiltrated the food supply. Those currently available include aspartame (NutraSweet, Equal), saccharin (Sweet'N Low, Sugar Twin), sucralose (Splenda), acesulfame-K (Sweet One, Sunett), and stevia (Truvia, Pure Via). Artificial sweeteners are regulated by the Food and Drug Administration and are generally recognized as safe. One downside to artificially sweetened foods, however, is that they are generally highly processed and devoid of healthful nutrients. Given the lack of benefit to consuming them, I'd play it safe and limit them to a serving or two a day in case scientists discover something harmful about them in the future. Why make a guinea pig out of yourself?

Two Approaches for Managing Carbs

The prediabetes diet plan offers two approaches for managing the amount of carbohydrate you're eating: the balanced-plate approach and the carb-counting approach (these are detailed in chapters 4 and 5). Which method you prefer depends on whether you're more comfortable (at least in the beginning) with making more general changes or if you prefer a more con-trolled approach of working within a specific carb budget at each meal or snack. My personal preference is to start with broader changes, knowing you can always tighten things up as time goes on and you become more confident in your ability to read labels and manage your portions.

The balanced-plate approach works well for a lot of people just getting started, because they can focus on simple strategies that shift carb intake to a lower level made up of better-quality choices. For others who perhaps are more into numbers, or who need some hard-core boundaries on carb intake to help with portion control, there's the carb-counting approach. Both methods can result in good control of carbohydrate and calorie intake. There is no right or wrong between the two. I embrace a start-out-small approach that only needs to get as complicated as my clients want it to.

Regardless of the method you choose, spreading carbs out into smaller portions throughout the day is critical to the success of the prediabetes diet plan. When you eat carbs, within an hour the majority have been digested and released as glucose into your blood. The goal of these carb-distributed plans is to maintain a sustained blood glucose level that fluxes within a steady range—not too high, not too low—so your blood glucose levels are rolling like hills rather than widely varying in a mountains-and-valleys pattern. When you eat a moderate amount of carbs at once, you get a more muted insulin release that reduces the pancreas's workload and should help bring glucose levels back to baseline without overshooting the mark (and causing sensations of low blood sugar and subsequent hunger). With a large load of carbs eaten at once, you'll respond with a more aggressive insulin surge, which will lower your blood glucose levels—possibly too much—causing sensations of low blood sugar and subsequent cravings for carbs as a means of restocking blood glucose levels to a steady state.

Taking all that into account, it makes sense that if you eat a breakfast that's lower in carbohydrate than it has been, you may also like to have a fruit or some other small portion of carbohydrate (with or without a small amount of protein) midmorning to keep yourself from becoming overhungry by lunch. Lunch and dinner are usually significantly farther apart, so a planned protein and carb snack (with something you bring to the office from home, which is generally a healthier choice) eaten midafternoon (when you're maybe a little hungry but not starving) can go a long way toward preventing extreme hunger and subsequent overeating. If you don't want to overeat, you need to eat frequently enough to help keep your hunger in check. And that takes forethought and planning. As we move on to chapter 4, we'll start with the balanced-plate approach. Chapter 5 covers the carb-counting method. Whether you ever get to this more advanced number-crunching part of the prediabetes diet plan is entirely your choice.

4

Building a Balanced Plate: Carb-Distributed Diet Approach 1

The balanced-plate approach focuses on restructuring how different kinds of foods populate your plate based on their carbohydrate content. This method is similar to those of other organizations, including the USDA's ChooseMyPlate.gov, which replaced the Food Pyramid with the plate approach; the American Institute for Cancer Research's New American Plate for cancer prevention; and the Harvard School of Public Health's Healthy Eating Plate—all of which are designed to promote a healthier weight, better heart health, and a lower risk of diabetes and cancer.[1] There are multiple health benefits to be reaped from this approach.

Contrary to the typical American diet—where half the plate is protein, like meat or chicken, or half the plate is starch from rice, potato, or pasta—with the balanced-plate approach, half the plate is nonstarchy vegetables.

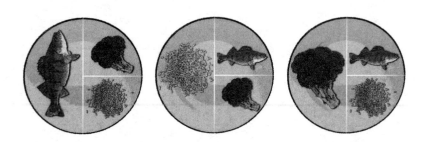

The idea is to manage what's on your plate so you're visually satisfied and don't feel deprived, but the net effect of what happens in your bloodstream and metabolism is conducive to lowering your circulating insulin levels and trimming calories from your diet. Let's break down the balanced-plate approach into steps, including what to eat and why.

Balanced Plate: Step 1

Cover half your plate with nonstarchy vegetables. What's so great about this veggie-heavy approach? First, plate size matters. Studies show that bigger plates encourage bigger portions. In the 1980s plates averaged ten inches in diameter, but today plates average twelve inches across, never mind the much larger square and rectangular platters that are so big some people report not being able to fit them into their cabinets! Dinner plates a century ago were the size of modern-day salad plates, so try packing away your dinner plates and opt for salad plates as your standard dinnerware. They may also serve as a reminder to start your meal with a filling salad loaded with low-calorie, nutrient-rich vegetables. If you then eat your main meal off the same plate, it will also save on after-dinner cleanup!

One of the main purposes of covering half your plate with vegetables is to help take up space in your stomach with foods that are low in carbohydrates and calories because they're mostly water. Part of what contributes to the biological process of feeling full is that as your stomach stretches out, chemicals are released into your system, stimulating that feeling of fullness. If you don't have any vegetables on your plate, by default you'll be relying on more calorie-dense foods—like meat, chicken, cheese, bread, pasta, rice, and potatoes—to do all the stretching. You want less room on your plate—and in your stomach—for carb- and calorie-rich food. Covering half your plate with vegetables is healthy for loads of reasons: not only will it help you lose weight and blunt your insulin response, it will also lower your risk of heart disease, cancer, and many other chronic health problems.

Vegetables can be cooked, raw, or served in a soup or salad. Eating more does require planning how and where you're going to fit them in. Start your meal with a salad with low-fat dressing, which may help fill you up and blunt your appetite, and follow it up with one or two cooked vegetables. Broth-based vegetable soup makes for a good meal starter. Filling up on this mostly water food at the beginning of a meal may help reduce your intake of the more calorie-dense foods served later. Homemade soup is one of the easiest things to prepare in bulk, even if you just make it up as you go along, using a premade broth, frozen vegetables, and a can of kidney beans. When choosing vegetables, include a variety of colors. Besides diversifying your intake of vitamins and minerals, many of the health-promoting phytonutrients in plants are the same compounds that give a plant its pigment. Varying color varies phytonutrients, so if you find you're always eating green vegetables, for example, throw in some red, yellow, orange, purple, and white ones to mix up your phytonutrients.

If you haven't been a vegetable eater, now is the time to start retrying all those vegetables you assume you don't like, to see if your taste has changed. Just because you didn't like something earlier in life doesn't mean you still won't like it, particularly if it's prepared in a more contemporary way. Taste does change over time, but you'll never know if you don't take a chance. Try different vegetables raw, steamed, roasted, sautéed in olive oil and garlic, tossed in lemon juice or balsamic vinegar, mixed into a soup, on top of a pizza, or grilled on the barbecue. There are bound to be some vegetables you like if you keep an open mind. Don't assume you'll hate something before you try it.

Take advantage of opportunities to try something new, such as when eating at a friend's house or dining out. Take a trip to a farm stand or produce market where sellers often share tips and recipes on how to prepare their foods. I'd never eaten brussels sprouts until several years ago when I had some roasted while dining out. I couldn't believe how delicious they were, and we've been cooking them at home ever since. It's not that I thought I wouldn't like them, I'd just never given them much thought.

Balanced Plate: Step 2

Cover about 25 percent of your plate with lean protein, including some plant sources. If there's one thing we learned from the low-carb craze, it's that protein is important. It slows the rate at which food leaves your stomach, lending a greater feeling of fullness to a meal. Think about it: How long does a salad with fat-free dressing last you before you feel hungry again? What if you add some grilled chicken, a hard-boiled egg, or some beans (or a bit of all three)? Including protein on your plate definitely holds hunger at bay for longer. Because the same fats that are bad for your heart (saturated and trans fats) may worsen insulin resistance, it's important to pick lean sources of protein. These include the following:

- Chicken or turkey breast (not fried)
- Fish and seafood (not fried)
- Lean meat (anything with the words "loin," "round," or "flank" in the name, or 90 percent lean or leaner)
- Tofu, tempeh, and other foods made with soy, like veggie burgers, tofu dogs, and TVP (textured vegetable protein)
- Beans, such as kidney beans, lentils, chickpeas (garbanzos), white beans (cannellini), black beans, and pinto beans

Soy foods and beans also count as carbohydrates, and they are good sources of dietary fiber, which helps to blunt the postmeal glucose response. It makes sense, however, to keep an eye on the other sources of carbs in the meal (one of the unique challenges for vegetarians). Beyond hunger and glucose/insulin control, protein is important to the body for many reasons and is often neglected, particularly by women trying to lose weight who may view protein foods as "fattening."

Balanced Plate: Step 3

Cover the remaining 25 percent of your plate with a healthy starch choice, such as a whole grain or starchy vegetable. During the low-carb years, all types of carbs, including fruit, which most people intuitively know is good for you, were deemed bad because "they contain too much sugar." But eating specific foods doesn't make you fat. Eating too many calories and not burning them off is what causes weight gain over time. High-quality starch choices include brown or wild rice, whole wheat pasta, quinoa, or whole grain breads. Starchy vegetables include potatoes, sweet potatoes, yams, winter squash, peas, corn, and beans, such as kidney or garbanzo beans. Allotting one-fourth of a medium-sized plate takes care of the quantity as long as you abstain from seconds! If that portion size still seems vague, take your knowledge a step further by learning how to count carbohydrates (see chapter 5).

Balanced Plate: Step 4

Include a dab of healthy fat to enhance the flavor and add some healthful nutrients. The balanced plate accounts for the carbohydrate, protein, and nonstarchy vegetable part of the meal. But what about the fat? Including some fat enhances the flavor and texture, helps with absorption of fat-soluble nutrients (vitamins A, D, E, and K as well as many phytonutrients), helps foods brown during cooking, and generally makes food taste good! The key is to mind the Two Qs (quality and quantity). The fats of the heart-healthy Mediterranean diet (like olive oil, canola oil, nuts, seeds, and avocados) are good for you. But when it comes to calories, fat is fat. Whether it's heart-healthy olive oil or butter, it's still 120 calories per tablespoon. What is a reasonable amount of fat? Try limiting it to two servings per meal. The following is a list of what counts as a serving of fat:

- 1 teaspoon vegetable oil (preferably olive, canola, or peanut), butter, or tub margarine (trans fat–free only)
- 1 tablespoon light margarine (trans fat–free only)
- 1 tablespoon seeds (sesame, pumpkin, or flaxseeds)
- ⅓ ounce nuts (for specifics, see the sidebar "Nuts: An Important Caveat" on page 91)
- 1 tablespoon pine nuts
- 1½ teaspoons nut butter
- 2 teaspoons tahini (sesame paste)
- 2 teaspoons mayonnaise
- 1 tablespoon reduced-fat mayonnaise
- 1 tablespoon regular salad dressing
- 2 tablespoons reduced-fat salad dressing
- 8 olives
- 2 tablespoons of avocado

Remember, the recommended two servings include both fats used in cooking and fats added to foods at the table. Nuts, olives, and avocado are great additions to a salad (which likely also has dressing on), but you need to watch the quantity. One advantage to cooking at home is that you can control the amount of fat you use.

Mealtime Extras

As you can see, we haven't accounted for fruit, milk, and yogurt on our balanced plate, but you still need to pay attention to their carbohydrate content. The simple approach is to limit fruit intake to one serving at a time and to choose either an eight-ounce glass of milk or soy beverage, or a six- to eight-ounce yogurt at a meal or snack, not both. It is possible to mix and match carbs so things aren't this cut and dried, but in my experience it works well to aim for two to three servings of whole fruit daily but spread out over the day so you're eating only one at a time. (A serving of fruit is roughly the size of a tennis ball. For exact portions of different fruits, see the fruit list on page 81). That way your body has only one fruit's worth of sugar to deal with in the hours after your meal or snack.

It's okay to stop right here with the balanced-plate approach and not move on to counting carbs. But if you're ready to wade in for more specifics, or feel you need them to manage your portions, read on. Even if you decide not to count every gram of carbohydrate you eat, the lists of carb-containing foods will help you figure out what foods you should be limiting portions of on your balanced plate.

Mind-Set Intervention:
Don't Let Sabotaging Thoughts Sideline You

Some of you may be skeptical that a diet that's not highly structured can be effective. Over the years I've had countless requests from clients who feel they need to be told exactly what to eat every day, or feel they'll find a way to blow it and fail yet again. My response is this: "Have superstructured diets worked for you in the past? Were you able to make changes you could live with long term?" Usually the answer is no, but if some aspects of your structured plan worked well in the past, you should take those elements and incorporate them into the new habits you'll need to make permanent change. But you need to let go of the idea of forever eating off a meal plan. Remember the 80/20 rule: if most of the time you're eating pretty well and exercising, there should be some wiggle room in your eating plan. There's only so much food restricting you can do before you'll be hungry all the time, get frustrated, and eventually quit.

5

Carbohydrate Counting: Carb-Distributed Diet Approach 2

How much carbohydrate should you eat to meet your body's needs without overrestricting the healthy carbs that will do you good? The best way to figure this out is to estimate your calorie needs and then assess how much of that should come from carbohydrate. With insulin resistance, you'll want around 45 percent of your total daily calories to come from carbs. None of this discussion is designed to make you obsessed with numbers, but rather to give you an idea of what a reasonable amount of carbohydrate is, *for you*, and how to best consume that over the day.

Crunching the Numbers

There are simple ways to estimate your calories, the most user friendly being resources available on the Internet. Many online calorie estimators exist that will ask your age, weight, height, sex, and activity level and then estimate your calorie needs for maintenance of your current weight or for weight loss if that's your goal. For example, visit the USDA's ChooseMyPlate.gov and hit the tab for the SuperTracker, where you can plan, analyze, and track your diet and physical activity. You can also look up individual foods to see or compare their nutritional value, find recommendations for what and how much you should eat, compare your food choices to these recommendations and to your nutrient needs, and assess personal physical activities and how to improve.[1] To get started, you must first create a profile by entering your personal data (age, sex, height, weight, and average activity level) into the SuperTracker tool. Your profile will then outline a calorie level and food plan for maintaining your weight. If you'd like to lose weight, visit the "My Weight Manager" page, where you can enter in a goal weight and the program will recalculate your calorie level and meal plan for success. SuperTracker allows you to set up to five goals related to weight, calories, physical activity, food groups, and nutrients—your progress toward these goals will be reported back to you as you log your food and activity into the website. It takes some time to learn how to use the program, but once you've got it down, it can be a very helpful tool.

Online and smartphone applications abound in the arena of tracking calorie intake and physical activity. Popular websites and apps include MyFitnessPal.com, Lose It!, and the American Cancer Society's Calorie Counter Calculator, to name just a few.[2] Given the industry that's rising up around managing the obesity epidemic, new (and always improving) nutrition feedback and tracking programs are coming out fast and furious these days. See the Resources section at the back of the book for more on the many options available that can assist you with tracking your nutrition and weight-loss goals.

If you prefer the old-fashioned longhand way of crunching out your calories, you can also use the Mifflin St. Jeor equation, used by nutrition professionals to estimate calorie needs in both healthy normal-weight and obese adults.[3] The equation estimates resting calorie needs, on top of which you need to add average physical activity. You will definitely need a calculator. Here's how it works:

First, calculate your basal metabolic rate (BMR), which tells you how many calories you burn at rest just keeping yourself alive (basically the caloric cost of keeping your heart beating, breathing, digesting food, maintaining your muscles and other organs, and so on). Like most scientific equations, the Mifflin St. Jeor uses metric measurements, so you'll need to calculate your weight in kilograms (kg) and your height in centimeters (cm). Here's how you do it: 1 kg = 2.2 pounds, so a 150-pound person weighs 68 kg. Also, 1 inch = 2.54 cm, so a 6-foot-tall person (72 inches) is approximately 183 cm. It's okay to round up or down to the nearest kilogram or centimeter.

Now that you know your weight and height in metrics, let's crunch some numbers:

For women: BMR = (10 × weight in kg) + (6.25 × height in cm) – (5 × age) – 161

For men: BMR = (10 × weight in kg) + (6.25 × height in cm) – (5 × age) + 5

Once you've calculated your BMR, you need to multiply that number by an "activity factor," which adds on additional calories for activity:[4]

- Sedentary, meaning little to no physical activity = 1.2
- Light activity up to three times a week = BMR × 1.375
- Moderate activity three to five times a week = BMR × 1.55
- Vigorous activity six to seven times a week = BMR × 1.725
- Extreme activity, such as intense sports training six to seven days a week = BMR × 1.9

Let's run through an example, using a thirty-five-year-old woman who weighs 185 pounds and is 5 feet 7 inches tall:

(10 × weight of 84 kg) + (6.25 × height of 170 cm) – (5 × 35) – 161 = 1,566 calories for BMR. Her current activity is light, so we take her BMR of 1,566 calories × 1.375 = 2,153 calories. Remember, this number is to maintain her current weight. But what if she wants to lose weight? The conventional wisdom is that if you want to aim for about one pound of weight loss per week, you should trim 500 calories from your diet, based on the rough assumption that a pound of body fat is equal to about 3,500 calories, so eating 500 fewer calories for seven days theoretically should result in a one-pound loss of body fat. But do understand that the mathematical estimates of how much weight you should lose aren't perfect. Not everyone will lose a pound per week if they eat 500 fewer calories per day. We each have our own unique genetics and physiology that can affect calorie balance. The best we can do is estimate calories needed for weight loss and fine-tune things as we go along.

For many of us, cutting 500 calories is too extreme, though—our brains would definitely notice an absence of 500 calories, possibly ramping up our preoccupation with food. A better alternative—and one that recognizes the mandatory contribution of regular physical activity to weight loss—is to trim about 200 to 250 calories from your diet and add in an equal amount of calories burned through physical activity. If you're really stressed about cutting calories and want to take things slower, cut even fewer calories and get serious with the exercise. You'll likely still lose a little weight, but eventually you'll hit a plateau where you stop losing. At this point, you may be ready to trim more calories. Research suggests that you can reduce your food intake by about 20 percent and still fly below the radar of that primitive monitoring system in your brain that will ramp up your preoccupation with food if it thinks you're eating too little.[5]

Again, it's better to go slow and steady, focusing on making permanent changes that can stick, rather than cutting a lot of calories and losing weight fast, only to regain it "with interest" when your ability to tolerate the drastic change burns out. No calorie calculator can take into account body composition. There will always be people who weigh more because they have more lean muscle, which only very expensive, high-tech body composition analysis machines will be able to figure out. Rest assured, however, that most of us do not fall into this category!

Calculating Carbs from Calories

Once you've calculated your total calorie needs, to figure out the calories that should come from carbohydrates, and then the grams, take your total calorie number and multiply it by 0.45 (because we're aiming for 45 percent of your daily calories to come from carbs). (Your registered dietitian may recommend a different percentage of calories from carbohydrate, which you can easily adjust for by changing the multiplier. For example, for 50 percent of calories from carb, multiply your base calorie number by 0.50 instead of 0.45.) This is a rough estimate of the number of calories you should eat from carbohydrates per day. For example, say your estimated needs are 2,000 calories a day. Take 2,000 × 0.45 = 900 carb calories. Food labels don't list carb calories, though; they list grams. There are 4 calories per gram of carbohydrate, so if you take that 900 and divide it by 4, you'll get your total grams of carbohydrate per day, which in this example would be 225 grams. Remember that this amount of carbohydrate will be divided over three meals and at least one or two snacks. If you look at any food label large enough to list the recommended daily values from total fat, saturated fat, cholesterol, sodium, total carbohydrate, and dietary fiber, they are based on a 2,000-calorie diet. This is referred to as the "footnote" of the Nutrition Facts label and appears at the bottom of the chart on the following page.

Nutrition Facts

Serving Size 1 slice
Servings Per Container 20

Amount Per Serving

Calories 90	Calories from Fat 15

	% Daily Value*
Total Fat 2g	3%
Saturated Fat 0g	0%
Trans Fat 0g	
Cholesterol 0mg	0%
Sodium 130mg	5%
Total Carbohydrate 15g	5%
Dietary Fiber 2g	8%
Sugars 1g	
Protein 4g	

Vitamin A 0%	Vitamin C 0%	
Calcium 4%	Iron 4%	

Percent daily value reflects "as packaged" food.

* Percent daily values are based on a 2,000 calorie diet. Your daily values may be higher or lower depending on your calorie needs:

	Calories:	2,000	2,500
Total Fat	Less than	65g	80g
Sat Fat	Less than	20g	25g
Cholesterol	Less than	300mg	300mg
Sodium	Less than	2,400mg	2,400mg
Total Carbohydrate		300g	375g
Dietary Fiber		25g	30g
Calories per gram:	Fat 9	Carbohydrate 4	Protein 4

The recommended daily value for carbohydrate based on a 2,000-calorie diet is 300 grams per day. My calculation for someone with insulin resistance recommends an allowance of about 225 grams of carb per day. This is 25 percent below the usual recommendation for carbs at this calorie level, but it is not a "low-carb" diet. Compare this to the 25 grams of carbs a day that are recommended during the "induction" phase of the Atkins diet. Many lost weight on this diet in the short term, but many reported problems with weakness, headaches, and serious irritability when they subjected their brain and nervous system to so little carbohydrate. Long term, it's neither healthy nor realistic to stick to consuming so little carbohydrate. How many people actually thought they could live out the rest of their lives without ever eating bread or pasta? Also, although the protein- and fat-dense foods touted in the Atkins plan were music to the ears of many, in the words of one of my patients: "I never thought I could get sick of the taste of bacon!"

Planning Meals and Snacks Within Your Carb Budget

Once you have your carb budget figured out, you need to determine how to best distribute them over the day. If, like the example above, you come up with 225 grams of carb, it's not going to help if you decide to divide them into two huge meals that are roughly 112 grams each. This large load of carbohydrate eaten at one sitting will result in a pretty large bolus of glucose released into your blood an hour later, with a subsequent hefty release of insulin into your system. Assuming a healthier eating pattern of three meals a day, a much more reasonable amount of carbohydrate to consume at one meal is in the range of 45 to 60 grams per meal for women and 60 to 75 grams per meal for men (women may also fall into this range if they're tall or very active).

Aiming for a carb range at meals and snacks is a good thing. It prevents you from obsessing about a specific number and allows for some flexibility. Given that carbohydrates yield 4 calories per gram, 45 grams of carbohydrate is 180 calories, 60 grams is 240 calories, and 75 is 300 calories. So whether you should aim for 45, 60, or 75 grams of carb largely depends on how much you're trying to control your calories (the calories from the protein and fat you're eating count toward the total for your meal as well) and how hungry you are at the moment.

Where Those with Diabetes Have the Edge

Someone who has diabetes can figure out how much carbohydrate they should be eating based on what their individual postmeal glucose response is. Both the American Diabetes Association and the American College of Endocrinology make recommendations for what blood glucose levels should be two hours after a meal and suggest that a reading of less than 180 mg/dl is good and less than 140 mg/dl is better.[6] How much carbohydrate someone with diabetes can get away with eating and still hit this goal can vary—maybe 45 grams, maybe 60 grams, maybe 75 or even higher. Those with diabetes can actually see what their body thinks of what they just ate. If it was too much carbohydrate, their blood glucose will be too high after a meal. They can then adjust down their carb intake the next time they eat a similar meal—maybe switch to light bread, move the fruit out of the meal and into a snack later on, or eat a smaller portion of dessert.

Let's construct a daily meal plan based on our sample carb budget of 225 grams.

Daily Meal Plan 1

Breakfast	60 grams
Lunch	60 grams
Dinner	60 grams
Total	**180 grams**

We've used up 180 grams of our 225-gram budget at meals. That leaves 45 grams of carb left to distribute between meals and snacks. Here's one way to do it:

Daily Meal Plan 2

Breakfast	60 grams
Midmorning snack	15 grams
Lunch	60 grams
Afternoon snack	30 grams
Dinner	60 grams
Total	**225 grams**

Another way to spread the carbs out over the day could look like this:

Daily Meal Plan 3

Breakfast	60 grams
Midmorning snack	15 grams
Lunch	60 grams
Afternoon snack	15 grams
Dinner	60 grams
Evening snack	15 grams
Total	**225 grams**

How might this be different if you were aiming for a lower intake, like 1,600 calories? Let's crunch the numbers: 1,600 calories × 0.45 = 720 carbohydrate calories. Divide 720 by 4 calories per gram for carbohydrates = 180 grams total carbs for the day. With this lower calorie goal, assume 45 grams of carbohydrate per meal:

Daily Meal Plan 4

Breakfast	45 grams
Lunch	45 grams
Dinner	45 grams
Total	**135 grams**

This leaves us with 45 grams of carb to spread between meals as snacks:

Daily Meal Plan 5

Breakfast	45 grams
Midmorning snack	15 grams
Lunch	45 grams
Afternoon snack	30 grams*
Dinner	45 grams
Total	**180 grams**

*Note: A 1,400-calorie meal plan would look similar, only the afternoon snack would be 15 grams of carbohydrate instead of 30 grams.

Think of your carb budget per meal as money to spend—if you only have seventy-five dollars in your wallet, you can't buy a pair of shoes that cost one hundred dollars! Of course, we haven't factored in the protein and fat calories yet, and all calories count when it comes to losing weight. Once you start being mindful of eating according to a regular meal pattern, prioritizing eating your next meal or snack before you're starving—along with quelling your insulin response by curbing the amount of carbs you eat at a meal or snack—it will be easier not to eat too much food. You just won't crave it as much.

Using Carb Counting to Learn Healthy Portions

For some people, simply eating off a smaller plate and following the balanced-plate approach is enough to help curb carb and calorie intake. For those who need a little more guidance to control their portion of starch—or feel completely clueless about the amount of carbohydrate in the foods they're used to eating—carb counting helps set limits. For decades those with diabetes have been using the *Diabetes Exchange Lists for Meal Planning*, published by the American Diabetes Association.[7] Here foods are grouped together into lists of similar foods—starches, fruits, milk/yogurt, sweets/desserts, vegetables, proteins, and fats. Our focus is on the first four lists—starches, fruits, milk/yogurt, and sweets/desserts—because those are the ones that provide significant sources of carbs.

Most vegetables contain very little carbohydrate per serving, as they're mostly water and fiber, which is indigestible carbohydrate that doesn't show up as sugar in your blood after digestion. The vegetable list contains veggies with so little carb per serving that I consider them a "free food." (The ADA exchange lists say that three servings of nonstarchy vegetables count as a carb choice, but for our purposes they're free in any amount. In all my years of nutrition counseling, I've yet to see a client overdo it on salad and broccoli.) Starchy vegetables (potatoes, corn, and peas) and a few other foods are listed in the starch list. Protein foods do not contain carbs, and even though they require some insulin for processing, the effect is not significant. Choices in this group are listed according to fat and calorie content (because of the need to follow a heart healthy diet and control calories), and lean sources of protein are encouraged. Fats are also listed according to how heart healthy they are. Saturated and trans fats are discouraged, and monounsaturated and omega-3 fats encouraged. Like protein foods, even though these foods don't require insulin for processing, whether a fat is heart healthy or not, all fats provide a lot of calories in a small serving, so portion control is key.

Within each list, this system of tracking carbs breaks foods down into portions that would provide a similar amount of carbohydrate, using 15 grams of carbohydrate per portion as the standard reference. A budget of 45 to 75 grams of carb per meal and 15 to 30 grams of carb per snack includes all the carbohydrate foods added together—grains, fruit, starchy

Mind-Set Intervention: Don't Stress About the Numbers

Some people get freaked out or overwhelmed by numbers. That's why I always start with the balanced-plate approach and build on that if people appear ready for counting carbs. You can pick and choose whether, or to what degree, you want to count carbohydrate grams, calories, or anything else. Some people feel they need to count carb grams to get a grip on what a portion of carbohydrate really looks like. Others just like the sense of having a carb goal for a meal or snack so they can recognize a good carb snack choice from reading the label or to help them make sense of a combination food, like pizza, for example: one slice of a fourteen-inch hand-tossed Dominos pizza is 37 grams of carbohydrate. Hang up the perfectionism here, and read on with an open mind.

vegetables, milk, yogurt, and sweets. Each carb-containing food is worth 15 grams, and you decide how many of these choices you're going to use at a meal or snack. You can decide which carbs you want to eat and estimate how much you can eat from each source (i.e., each food list) to keep within your carb budget for that meal or snack. The rest of the calories for your meals and snacks are filled in with nonstarchy vegetables, lean protein choices, and moderate amounts of healthy fats. Chapter 6 delves much deeper into the specifics of the exchange lists.

6

The Details of Counting Carbohydrates

For many people, the balanced-plate approach provides an easy-to-understand visual of what should be on their plate. Covering half your plate with nonstarchy vegetables is pretty straightforward. That means aiming to eat more vegetables than you probably have been eating. A portion of cooked protein that's somewhere between the size of a deck of cards (three ounces) and a hockey puck (four ounces)—maybe a little more if you're a man—is something we can relate to. The toughest foods to control portions of are often the starches (grains and starchy vegetables, like potatoes), the very foods you want to be paying attention to here, as well as the amount of fat we eat, particularly if you dine out a lot. Make sure you spread out the carbohydrate you get from fruit, milk or yogurt, and sweets, and consider their nutritional contribution to a total meal or snack.

Just as counting calories and fat grams are strategies to help manage your diet, carbohydrate counting is designed to help you get a grip on portions. The main difference is that with keeping track of fat grams or calories, we don't think so much about how they are being distributed over the day; instead, we focus on the daily total. With carb counting, however, we're trying to control the glucose/insulin response that occurs immediately after each meal and snack, so it's as much about the distribution as it is about the numbers.

Back to the Numbers

In chapter 5 we outlined how to calculate calories for the day and how to use that number to calculate your daily carb budget. Breaking that down into meals and snacks leaves most people with 45 to 75 grams of carbohydrate per meal and 15 to 30 grams per snack. All other foods being the same, 45 grams per meal and 15 grams per snack will save you some calories over the plan of 60 to 75 grams of carb per meal and 30 grams per snack. For most people with prediabetes, weight loss is a part of their plan. Losing weight is about eating fewer calories (and burning more through activity). Eating fewer calories requires portion control, which is much easier if you stay ahead of your hunger by eating a reasonably sized meal or snack every three to four hours. If we look back at the balanced-plate idea, what you're trying to do is control the amount of starch on that quarter of the plate while keeping an eye on how many other carb foods you'll be eating with the meal. For decades many people with diabetes have been using the American Diabetes Association (ADA) *Exchange Lists for Diabetes* to get a grip on carb serving sizes.[1] With this system, similar foods are grouped together:

- Starches
- Fruits
- Milk and yogurt
- Sweets, desserts, and other carbohydrates
- Nonstarchy vegetables
- Meat and meat substitutes
- Fats

The exchange lists break down foods into groups based on the three major nutrients: carbohydrates, proteins (meat and meat substitutes), and fats. Each list contains foods grouped together based on similar nutrient content. They are called "exchange lists" because each food is listed according to the serving size that would provide roughly the same amount of carbohydrate, protein, fat, and calories in a portion. It may be easier to think of these servings as carbohydrate food choices, aiming for a certain number per meal or snack. For carb-containing foods, the serving sizes are determined by the amount of that food that contains 15 grams of carbohydrate. You can "exchange" one serving of food within the same list for another and expect the same blood sugar rise, and subsequent insulin response, regardless of which food you choose. As part of the prediabetes diet plan, the main focus of the exchange lists is primarily on the first three lists—the starches, fruits, and milk/yogurt—because these are the

Eat Your Beans

Under no circumstances should you use the fact that beans contain carbs as a reason not to eat them. They are one of the highest-fiber foods you can eat, providing both soluble and insoluble fiber; they are a great source of plant protein; and they are a source of many other important nutrients, such as iron, B vitamins, magnesium, and potassium. Studies show that eating more plant protein may help with weight management and lower your risk of many chronic diseases.[2] One cup of kidney beans has 37 grams of carbohydrate, but 13 of those grams are fiber, which is indigestible and slows down the release of glucose into your blood. So eat beans—every day if you can, even if it's only in small quantities thrown into a soup or tossed into a salad, or as a couple of tablespoons of hummus.

significant sources of carbs. The exchange lists also provide estimates on reasonably sized servings of sweets. Let's take a look at each group.

Starch. The starch list includes breads, cereals, rice, pasta, crackers, starchy snack foods, and other types of nontraditional whole grains, such as quinoa, barley, couscous, and bulgur. The starch list also includes starchy vegetables (vegetables whose sugar content would look more like bread than broccoli under a microscope), such as beans, peas, lentils, corn, potatoes, sweet potatoes, yams, winter squash, and plantains.

Fruit. The fruit list includes fresh fruit, canned fruit, dried fruit, and 100 percent fruit juice.

Milk. The milk list includes milk and yogurt. One percent (low-fat) and nonfat choices are encouraged.

Sweets, desserts, and other carbs. This list offers advice on how to work foods with added sugars into your plan by swapping out another carb source. Because sweets contain a large amount of carbohydrate in a small portion, the suggested portion sizes—like a 1¼-inch-square brownie or a 2-inch-square piece of chocolate cake—are radically small compared to what you might be used to, but that's all part of portion control.

Nonstarchy vegetables. The nonstarchy vegetables list includes most fresh, frozen, and canned vegetables as well as tomato and vegetable juices. These foods have so little carbohydrate per serving that I consider them a free food, as opposed to the starchy vegetables, which do need to be counted toward your daily distributed carb budget.

Meat and meat substitutes. This list includes animal sources of protein (meat, poultry, seafood, eggs, and cheese) as well as plant-based protein (beans, tofu, tempeh, soy nuts and edamame, nut butters, and other soy-based foods like veggie burgers, soy dogs, veggie nuggets and patties, and soy "crumbles"). Choices are separated into lean, medium-fat, high-fat, and plant-based choices. Animal sources of protein foods do not contain carbs, but many plant-based protein sources do, counting as both a protein and a carbohydrate. Plant-based proteins should be incorporated into your weekly meal plan. Just be sure to take into account what other sources of carbs you may also be eating at that meal (for example, eat less rice to make room for beans, which are a better source of carbohydrate anyway because they're loaded with fiber). Even though animal sources of protein require some insulin for processing, the effect is not significant. When paired with a carb, protein helps complicate digestion, slowing down the breakdown of carbs into glucose, thereby blunting your insulin response and leaving you with a more lasting feeling of fullness. Choices from animal sources in the protein group are listed according to fat and calorie content (because of the need to follow a heart-healthy diet and control calories). Lean sources of protein are encouraged.

Fats. This list includes oils, spreads, nuts and nut butters, seeds, olives, avocados, salad dressings, and mayonnaise. Choices are separated into heart-healthy monounsaturated, polyunsaturated, and omega-3 fats (encouraged) and unhealthy saturated and trans fats (limit or avoid). Like protein foods, even though fats don't require insulin for processing, they deliver a big calorie punch in a small serving, so portion control is key.

Alcohol. Alcohol is also addressed in the exchange lists. The ADA recommends limiting alcohol to one drink a day for women, two drinks a day for men. Up to this amount may be associated with some health benefits, although because of the potential negatives associated with alcohol use in some people, you should not start drinking alcohol solely for the health benefits. Be sure to factor in the calories if you're trying to lose weight. The following amounts constitute one drink:

- 12 ounces of beer
- 5 ounces of wine
- 1½ ounces of distilled spirits (80 proof)
- 1 ounce of coffee liqueur

A serving of beer is often clear because of its 12-ounce bottling, but many people can be heavy-handed when pouring wine and spirits. Test your hand with a liquid measuring cup so you know exactly how much you're consuming.

Free foods. The exchange lists include a section on foods that, when limited to the listed portion, will weigh you down with fewer than 20 calories and no more than 5 grams of carb per serving. This allows you to write off small portions of foods that contain sugar but simply don't add up to much when eaten in small amounts—things like a single hard candy, a tablespoon of ketchup, ¼ cup of salsa, or a couple of teaspoons of barbecue sauce.

Setting the Foundation for Carb Counting

Within each exchange list, the system breaks foods down into portions that would provide a similar amount of carbohydrate, using 12 to 15 grams of carb per portion as the reference serving size. A serving of starch or fruit has 15 grams of carbohydrate, and a serving of milk (any kind) or yogurt (plain or artificially sweetened, called "light" on the label) contains roughly 12 grams of carbohydrate. Because the difference between 12 and 15 grams of carb is so small, for simplicity's sake let's count a milk/yogurt serving as containing 15 grams of carbohydrate. Because the carb content of a serving of starch, fruit, or milk is basically the same, you can interchange a starch, a fruit, or milk at a meal or snack and consider them all one 15-gram carb choice.

Balance is important. To diversify your nutrients, you want to be eating carbs from different groups every day. Getting used to thinking of carbs in 15-gram choices fits into your budget of 45 grams (three choices), 60 grams (four choices), or 75 grams (five choices) of carb per meal, and 15 grams (one choice) to 30 grams (two choices) of carb per snack. (Remember: The category of 75 grams (five choices) per meal is generally reserved for those who are larger men or people who are really tall or active.) Thinking about carbohydrate foods in 15-gram carb servings allows you to look at any food label and determine how many carb serving "equivalents" there are in a serving of any food. For example, if a cereal label lists one serving as having 30 grams of carbohydrate, in your head you'll begin to recognize that as two carb choices.

Fiber is indigestible carbohydrate, so according to the American Diabetes Association, if the fiber content is 5 grams or more (of either soluble or insoluble fiber), you can subtract half that number from the total carbs listed on the label.[3] For example, if a cereal has 30 grams of carb in a serving, but 6 of it is fiber, then you "count" the serving as having 27 grams of carb (slightly less than two carb choices). Round up if that half number isn't even—for example, round 4.5 grams up to 5. Once you begin to view carbohydrates in 15-gram carb units, you can then decide which carbs you want to eat at a meal or snack and estimate how much you can eat of each food to keep within your per meal or snack carb budget. Keep in mind the benefits of pairing carbohydrates with protein and a little bit of healthy fat if possible (for example, a few whole grain crackers with reduced-fat cheese), to blunt the postmeal insulin response and help you stay feeling fuller longer. The 80/20 rule applies here as well: aim to pair your carbs with protein 80 percent of the time so that what happens the other 20 percent of the time doesn't matter as much.

By no means is carb counting meant to rationalize eating 60 grams of junk food carbs in place of food that does your body good. A 20-ounce soda has 65 grams of carbohydrate in it, but don't let such a processed, nutrient-poor food gobble up so much of your daily carb budget! If you're going to budget in some sweets, cut back a little on your healthy carbs to make room for a small amount of a special treat on occasion.

Practicing Portions in an Ever-Expanding World

To use the exchange list system to accurately estimate the amount of carbohydrate (and calories) you're eating, knowledge of portion sizes is critical. Do you know what a cup of cereal or ⅓ cup of cooked rice looks like? Outfit your kitchen with a set of dry measuring cups, a liquid measuring cup that holds up to 2 cups, and a set of measuring spoons. Inexpensive plastic versions are sold in most supermarkets, often in the baking goods section. Consider buying a food scale. Fancy, more expensive scales can be found in cooking stores, but a cheap $10 postage scale may work just as well.

Why the need for measuring devices? Because the exchange lists are portion specific, and most of us are horrible judges of gauging portion sizes. All around us portion sizes have been expanding. Even if you're over forty and remember when fast food burgers were the size of a kiddie meal, or a soda bottle was eight ounces, you may still be as prone as anyone to underestimating portion sizes. Don't guess: measure it. In fact, measure your foods a few times so that you can begin to accurately eyeball serving sizes. Then occasionally go back and measure again to see if your portion sizes have grown (known as "portion creep")—they often have.

Planning Your Plate

The following provides a reference for the seven exchange lists: starches; fruit; milk; sweets, desserts, and other carbs; nonstarchy vegetables; meat and meat substitutes; and fats. Remember, the first four groups are the ones you're focusing on to control your daily distributed carb intake. The last three groups are there to help you make healthy choices and control your calorie and fat intake. These are the foods that help you walk away from a meal feeling full without ramping up your insulin response.

Let the balanced-plate method guide you in planning the rest of the meal: load half your plate with nonstarchy vegetables because they are very low in calories and carbs but still help contribute to a feeling of fullness. The meat and meat substitutes list contains foods that should cover about 25 percent of your plate: you need protein for good health; it helps you feel full after a meal; and it doesn't require a significant amount of insulin for processing (be mindful of other carb choices at your meal if you opt for beans, peas, or hummus as a vegetarian protein source). Try to pick low-fat protein options most of the time because they're much lower in calories. Make heart-healthy choices from the fats list, and be aware of the recommended portion sizes. Avoid pouring olive oil freely from the bottle! You may unknowingly add hundreds of calories to your meal.

The Starch List

Starches include cereals, grains, pasta, breads, crackers, starchy vegetables, and many snack foods (like granola bars) as well as cooked beans, peas, and lentils. In general, one starch is equivalent to the following:

- ½ cup cooked cereal, grain, or starchy vegetable
- ⅓ cup cooked rice or pasta
- 1 ounce (30 grams by weight) bread product, such as one regular-size slice of bread
- ¾ to 1 ounce of most snack foods

Things to consider: A choice on the starch list has 15 grams of carbohydrate, 0 to 3 grams of protein, 0 to 1 grams of fat, and 80 calories. Choose low-fat starches as often as possible ("low fat" means no more than 3 grams of fat per serving). When choosing dense starches like bagels and large bread rolls, check how much they weigh. Each ounce *by weight* (30 grams) is one starch choice. The metric weight of a serving appears in parentheses after the serving size. Many bagels are 4 ounces—or four starch choices! An open handful is about 1 cup or 1 to 2 ounces of a snack food. For maximum health benefits, eat three or more servings of whole grains each day.

The Starch List

FOOD	SERVING SIZE
BREAD	
Bagel, large (about 4 ounces)	¼ bagel (1 ounce)
Biscuit, 2½-inch diameter	1
Bread	
Reduced calorie	2 slices
White, whole grain, pumpernickel, rye, unfrosted raisin	1 slice (1 ounce)
Chapati, small (6-inch diameter)	1
Cornbread, 1¾-inch cube	1 (1½ ounces)
English muffin	½ (1 ounce)
Hot dog or hamburger bun	½ (1 ounce)
Naan bread (8-inch diameter)	¼ piece
Pancake (4-inch diameter)	1

The Starch List, continued

FOOD	SERVING SIZE
Pita (6-inch diameter)	½ pita
Roll, small, plain	1 (1 ounce)
Stuffing, bread	⅓ cup (higher-fat choice)
Taco shell (5-inch diameter)	2 (higher-fat choice)
Tortilla, corn or flour (6 inch diameter)	1
Tortilla, flour (10-inch diameter)	⅓ tortilla
Waffle (4-inch square)	1 (opt for whole grain; higher-fat choice)
CEREALS AND GRAINS	
Barley, cooked	⅓ cup
Bran, dry	
Oat	¼ cup
Wheat	½ cup
Bulgur (cooked)	½ cup
Cereals	
Bran	½ cup
Cooked (oats, oatmeal)	½ cup
Puffed	1½ cups
Shredded wheat, plain	½ cup
Sugar coated	½ cup
Unsweetened, ready-to-eat	¾ cup
Couscous	⅓ cup
Granola	
Low fat	¼ cup
Regular	¼ cup (higher-fat choice)
Grits, cooked	½ cup
Kasha	½ cup
Millet, cooked	⅓ cup
Muesli	¼ cup
Pasta, cooked	⅓ cup
Polenta, cooked	⅓ cup
Quinoa, cooked	⅓ cup
Rice, white or brown, cooked	⅓ cup
Tabouli, prepared	½ cup
Wheat germ, dry	3 tablespoons
Wild rice, cooked	½ cup

The Starch List, continued

FOOD	SERVING SIZE
STARCHY VEGETABLES	
Cassava	⅓ cup
Corn	½ cup kernels or ½ large cob
Hominy, canned	¾ cup
Mixed vegetables with corn, peas, or pasta	1 cup
Parsnips	½ cup
Peas, green	½ cup
Plantain, ripe	⅓ cup
Potato	
Baked with skin	¼ large (3 ounces)
Boiled, all kinds	½ cup or ½ medium
French fried (oven baked)	1 cup (2 ounces)
Mashed with milk and fat	½ cup
Pumpkin, canned, no sugar added	1 cup
Spaghetti with pasta sauce	½ cup
Squash (winter, acorn, butternut)	1 cup
Succotash	½ cup
Yam, sweet potato, plain	½ cup
CRACKERS AND SNACKS	
Crackers	
Animal crackers	8
Graham crackers	3 (2½-inch squares)
Matzo	¾ ounce
Melba toast, about 2-inch by 4-inch piece	4 pieces
Oyster crackers	20
Round butter-type	6
Saltine-type	6
Sandwich-style, cheese or peanut butter filling	3
Whole wheat crisp breads	2–5 (¾ ounce)
Whole wheat regular	2–5 (¾ ounce)

The Starch List, continued

FOOD	SERVING SIZE
Popcorn	3 cups
Pretzels	¾ ounce
Rice cakes (4-inch diameter)	2
Snack chips	
Fat free or baked (tortilla, potato), baked pita chips	15 20 (¾ ounce)
Regular (tortilla, potato)	9–13 (¾ ounce)
BEANS, PEAS, AND LENTILS *(Note: The choices on this list count as one starch and one lean protein.)*	
Baked beans	⅓ cup
Beans, cooked (black, pinto, garbanzo, kidney, lima, navy, white)	½ cup
Lentils, cooked (brown, yellow, green)	½ cup
Peas, cooked (black eyed, split)	½ cup
Refried beans, canned (look for fat-free)	½ cup

The Fruit List

Fruit can be fresh, frozen, canned, or 100 percent fruit juice. The fruit on the bottom of a flavored yogurt cup does not count as a fruit! A serving of fruit is as follows:

- ½ cup canned fruit or fruit salad
- ⅓ to ½ cup unsweetened fruit juice
- 1 small fruit (4 ounces)
- 2 tablespoons dried fruit

Things to consider: A choice on the fruit list has 15 grams of carb, 0 protein, 0 fat, and 60 calories. Limit fruit juice to one serving or less per day, as juice has zero fiber and is not filling. Fresh fruit is preferable whenever possible. Aim for a minimum of two fruits daily, but eat them at different times to spread out the fruit sugar throughout the day. Think of dried fruit as something you sprinkle on or mix into something else—it's very easy to go overboard when eaten on its own. Avoid fruits that have been canned in heavy syrup. Look for canned fruits that say "extra light syrup," "no sugar added," or "juice packed."

The Fruit List

FRUIT	SERVING SIZE
Apple, unpeeled, small	1 (4 ounces)
Apples, dried	4 rings
Applesauce, unsweetened	½ cup
Apricots	
Canned	½ cup
Dried	8 halves
Fresh	4 whole
Banana, extra small	1 (4 ounces)
Blackberries	¾ cup
Blueberries	¾ cup
Cantaloupe, small	⅓ melon or 2 cups cubed
Cherries	
Sweet, canned	½ cup
Sweet, fresh	12
Dates	3
Dried fruits (blueberries, cherries, cranberries, mixed fruit, raisins)	2 tablespoons
Figs	
Dried	1½
Fresh	1½ large or 2 medium (3½ ounces)
Fruit cocktail	½ cup
Grapefruit	
Large	½ (11 ounces)
Sections, canned	¾ cup
Grapes, small	17 (3 ounces)
Honeydew melon	1 slice or 1 cup cubed (10 ounces)
Kiwi	1 (3½ ounces)
Mandarin oranges, canned	¾ cup
Mango, small	½ fruit (5½ ounces) or ½ cup
Nectarine, small	1 (5 ounces)
Orange, small	1 (6 ounces)
Papaya	½ fruit or 1 cup cubed (8 ounces)
Peaches	
Canned	½ cup
Fresh, medium	1 (6 ounces)

The Fruit List, continued

FRUIT	SERVING SIZE
Pears	
Canned	½ cup
Fresh, large	½ (4 ounces)
Pineapple	
Canned	½ cup
Fresh	¾ cup
Plums	
Canned	½ cup
Dried (prunes)	3
Small	2 (5 ounces)
Raspberries	1 cup
Strawberries	1¼ cups whole berries
Tangerines, small	2 (8 ounces)
Watermelon	1 slice or 1¼ cups cubed (13½ ounces)
JUICES	
Apple juice/cider	½ cup
Fruit juice blends, 100 percent juice	⅓ cup
Grape juice	⅓ cup
Grapefruit juice	½ cup
Orange juice	½ cup
Pineapple juice	½ cup
Prune juice	⅓ cup

The Milk List

This list includes milk and yogurt (cheese is on the protein list). In general, a serving is 1 cup of milk, 8 ounces of plain yogurt, or 6 ounces of flavored yogurt. Things to consider: One milk serving is 12 grams of carbohydrate, 8 grams of protein, and 0 to 8 grams of fat. To keep things easy, we're going to round one milk serving up to 15 grams of carb, to be consistent with our other two carb groups (starches and fruits). Opt for 1 percent (low-fat) or nonfat milk; 2 percent milk is only slightly lower in fat than whole milk. If 1 percent or nonfat milk seems too watered down for you, try one of the enhanced milks that add milk solids to provide a thicker mouthfeel. If your milk is flavored (like vanilla soy or almond milk, for example) and is not artificially sweetened, it will use up another one of your carb choices at that meal (remember to count the extra carbs). Yogurt, if flavored, should be artificially sweetened or it will also use up another one of your carb choices at that meal. Plain or flavored Greek yogurt is also a good choice as it tends to have less added sugar (and two to three times the protein content of regular yogurt).

The Milk List

FOOD	SERVING SIZE
Chocolate milk (sugar-free, fat-free, or 1 percent)	1 cup
Eggnog	½ cup
Evaporated milk	½ cup
Milk, buttermilk, goat's milk	1 cup
Fat-free or 1 percent low-fat milk	1 cup
Rice milk (fat-free or low-fat)	1 cup
Soy milk (unflavored)	1 cup
Yogurt, plain nonfat or 1 percent	8 ounces
Yogurt, flavored with artificial sweetener	6 ounces

The Sweets, Desserts, and Other Carbohydrates List

You can substitute a choice from this list for other carbs from the starch, fruit, or milk lists, even though these foods contain added sugars. Each carb choice here is 15 grams of carb. It's critically important to be portion conscious, however, as the carbs from sweets add up quickly. Set a goal of limiting sweets to special occasions, particularly if "just one" for you tends to lead to "many." For physiological reasons, the more you indulge in sweets, the more you'll want them. This list highlights how many carb choices are gobbled up by a pretty small serving. A teaspoon of table sugar contains only 4 grams of carbohydrate and 16 calories, so that amount added to your coffee may be something you can work in. For many, the added sugars in processed foods are the biggest problem.

The Sweets, Desserts, and Other Carbohydrates List

FOOD	SERVING SIZE	CARB CHOICES
BEVERAGES		
Energy drink	8 ounces	2 carbs
Fruit drink or lemonade	8 ounces	2 carbs
Hot chocolate (regular or sugar-free)	8 ounces	1 carb
Sports drink	8 ounces	1 carb
DESSERTS		
Brownie, small	1¼-inch square	1 carb
Cake		
Angel food, unfrosted	1 slice (1/12 of cake)	2 carbs
Frosted	2-inch square	2 carbs
Unfrosted	2-inch square	1 carb
Cookies		
Chocolate chip	2 (2½ inches across)	1 carb
Gingersnap	3 cookies	1 carb
Sandwich with creme filling	2 small	1 carb
Sugar-free	3 small or 1 large	1 carb
Vanilla wafer	5 cookies	1 carb
Cupcakes, frosted	1 small	2 carbs
Fruit cobbler	½ cup	3 carbs
Gelatin, regular	½ cup	1 carb (sugar-free gelatin is free)

The Sweets, Desserts, and Other Carbohydrates List, continued

FOOD	SERVING SIZE	CARB CHOICES
Pie		
Fruit (double crust)	1 slice (⅙ of 8-inch pie)	3 carbs
Pumpkin or custard	1 slice (⅙ of 8-inch pie)	1½ carbs
Pudding		
Regular	½ cup	2 carbs
Sugar-free	½ cup	1 carb
CANDY, SWEETS, SWEETENERS		
Candy, hard	3 pieces	1 carb
Candy bar, chocolate/peanut	2 "fun-size" bars (1 ounce)	1½ carbs
Chocolate "kisses"	5 pieces	1 carb
Fruit snacks, chewy	1 roll	1 carb
Fruit spread, 100 percent fruit	1½ tablespoons	1 carb
Honey	1 tablespoon	1 carb
Jam or jelly	1 tablespoon	1 carb
Sugar	1 tablespoon	1 carb
Syrup (chocolate, regular maple)	1 tablespoon	1 carb
Syrup, light	2 tablespoons	1 carb
CONDIMENTS AND SAUCES		
Barbecue sauce	3 tablespoons	1 carb
Cranberry sauce	¼ cup	1½ carbs
Salad dressing, fat-free, low fat, cream based	3 tablespoons	1 carb
Sweet-and-sour sauce	3 tablespoons	1 carb
DOUGHNUTS, MUFFINS, AND PASTRIES		
Banana nut bread	1-inch slice	2 carbs
Doughnut		
Glazed	3¼ inches across	2 carbs
Plain	1 medium	1½ carbs
Muffin (4 ounces)	¼ muffin	1 carb

The Sweets, Desserts, and Other Carbohydrates List, continued

FOOD	SERVING SIZE	CARB CHOICES
FROZEN DESSERTS		
Frozen pop	1	½ carb
Frozen yogurt, fat-free and regular	½ cup	1 carb
Fruit juice bars, 100 percent fruit juice	1 bar	1 carb
Ice cream		
Fat-free	½ cup	1½ carbs
Light and no sugar added	½ cup	1 carb
Regular	½ cup	1 carb (high in fat and calories)
Sherbet and sorbet	½ cup	2 carbs
GRANOLA BARS, MEAL REPLACEMENT BARS, TRAIL MIX		
Granola bar, regular or low fat	1 bar (1 ounce)	1½ carbs
Meal replacement bar	1 bar (2 ounces)	2 carbs
Trail mix	1 ounce	1 carb

The Nonstarchy Vegetables List

These vegetables are so low in carbohydrate that I consider them "free." Using the balanced-plate approach, your goal is to cover half the plate with nonstarchy vegetables, as they help fill you up without loading you down with carbs and calories. They also are among the most nutrient-rich foods out there. If eating this quantity of vegetables is new to you, start by covering just a third of your plate and work your way up. A serving of nonstarchy vegetables is ½ cup of cooked vegetables or vegetable juice or 1 cup of raw vegetables. Things to consider: A serving of nonstarchy vegetables contains only 5 grams of carb, 2 grams of protein, and 25 calories. Try to include at least ½ cup cooked or 1 cup raw vegetables with lunch, and 1 cup cooked or 2 cups raw vegetables with dinner. Look for a variety of colors in the vegetables you're eating. Varying the colors helps diversify the phytonutrients in your diet. Watch how much fat you add to your vegetables. Every teaspoon of butter, tub margarine, or oil adds 40 calories. And remember, corn, peas, potatoes, sweet potatoes, winter squash, and beans are on the starch list.

The Nonstarchy Vegetables List

Artichoke	Asparagus	Baby corn
Bamboo shoots	Beans (green, wax, Italian)	Bean sprouts
Beets	Borscht (hearty vegetable soup)	Broccoli
Brussels sprouts	Cabbage	Carrots
Cauliflower	Celery	Coleslaw (no dressing)
Cucumber	Eggplant	Green onions or scallions
Greens (collard, kale, mustard, turnip)	Hearts of palm	Jicama
Kohlrabi	Leeks	Lettuce, all varieties
Mixed vegetables (without corn, peas, or pasta)	Mung bean sprouts	Mushrooms
Okra	Onions	Pea pods
Peppers, all varieties	Radishes	Rutabaga
Sauerkraut	Spinach	Squash (summer, zucchini)
Swiss chard	Tomatoes	Tomato sauce (crushed tomatoes, no sugar added)
Tomato/vegetable juice	Turnips	Water chestnuts

The Meat and Meat Substitutes List

The key to eating a little more protein without eating too much unhealthful saturated fat is to opt for lean sources of protein. Because protein is found in so many different foods (in both animal and plant sources), serving sizes vary. Things to consider: In general, a protein choice has no carbs (unless it's a plant protein like beans or soy products or is served in a sweet marinade or sauce), 7 grams of protein, and 3 to 8 or more grams of fat. Calories per choice range from 45 to 100 calories or more per serving depending on fat content.

For meat, poultry, or seafood, a choice is 1 ounce cooked, but you would portion out 3 to 6 ounces or so at a meal. The size of a deck of cards is about 3 ounces; 4 ounces is about the size of a hockey puck. A snack may include one to two protein choices (1 to 2 ounces of protein). Protein choices can be lean (0–3 grams of fat per ounce), medium fat (4–7 grams of fat per ounce), high fat (more than 8 grams of fat per ounce), or plant based (the fat varies). Try to choose proteins with 5 grams of fat or fewer per ounce.

The only protein foods that contain carbs are the plant-based proteins. If, according to the food label, the amount of plant protein you're eating contains close to 15 grams of carb, count it as a carb and a protein but give yourself a little wiggle room if you're not diabetic. Choose poultry, seafood, or plant-based proteins whenever possible. If you eat red meat or pork, choose lean select or choice cuts that have the word "loin," "round," or "flank" in the name, or are 90 percent lean or leaner. Bake, roast, broil, grill, poach, steam, or boil your meats instead of frying, and trim off all visible fat. It's okay to stir-fry your dinner protein as this method of cooking should only require about 2 tablespoons of oil for the whole recipe.

The Meat and Meat Substitutes List

FOOD	SERVING SIZE
LEAN MEATS AND MEAT SUBSTITUTES (45 calories per ounce)	
Beef, lean cuts trimmed of fat	1 ounce
Cheese with 3 grams of fat per ounce	1 ounce
Cottage cheese	¼ cup
Egg substitutes	¼ cup
Egg whites	2
Fish, any kind (not fried)	1 ounce
Game: buffalo, venison, and so on	1 ounce
Lamb: chop, leg, or roast	1 ounce
Oysters	6 medium
Pork, lean: Canadian bacon, rib or loin chop/roast, ham, tenderloin	1 ounce
Poultry without the skin	1 ounce
Salmon, canned	1 ounce
Sardines, canned	2 small
Sausages with 3 grams of fat or less per ounce	1 ounce
Shellfish: clams, crab, lobster, scallops, shrimp	1 ounce
Tuna canned with water, drained	1 ounce
Veal: loin, chop, roast	1 ounce
MEDIUM-FAT MEAT AND MEAT SUBSTITUTES (75 calories per ounce)	
Beef: corned beef, ground beef, prime grades trimmed of fat (prime rib), short ribs	1 ounce
Cheeses with 4 to 7 grams of fat per ounce	1 ounce
Egg	1
Fish, fried	1 ounce
Lamb: ground, rib roast	1 ounce
Pork: cutlet, shoulder roast	1 ounce
Poultry: chicken with skin, fried chicken, ground turkey	1 ounce
Ricotta cheese	¼ cup
Sausage with 4 to 7 grams of fat per ounce	1 ounce
Veal, cutlet (no breading)	1 ounce
HIGH-FAT MEAT AND MEAT SUBSTITUTES (try to eat three or fewer servings per week; these are 100 calories or more per ounce)	
Bacon: pork, turkey	2 slices
Cheese: regular American, blue, Brie, Cheddar, hard goat, Monterey Jack, queso, and Swiss	1 ounce

The Meat and Meat Substitutes List, continued

FOOD	SERVING SIZE
Hot dog: beef, pork, or combination (10 per 1-pound package)	1
Hot dog: turkey, chicken (10 per 1-pound package)	1
Pork: ground, sausage, spareribs	1 ounce
Sandwich meats, processed, with 8 grams of fat or more: bologna, hard salami, pastrami	1 ounce
Sausage with 8 grams of fat or more per ounce: bratwurst, Carbrizo, Italian, knockwurst, smoked, summer	1 ounce
PLANT-BASED PROTEINS (these contain some carbohydrates but much of it is fiber; calories vary)	
Baked beans	⅓ cup
Beans, cooked: black, garbanzo, kidney, lima, navy, pinto, white	½ cup
"Beef" or "sausage" crumbles, soy based	2 ounces
"Chicken" nuggets, soy based	2 (1½ ounces)
Edamame	½ cup
Falafel (spiced chickpeas and wheat patties; 2-inch diameter)	3
Hot dog, soy based	1
Hummus	⅓ cup
Lentils, cooked: brown, green, or yellow	½ cup
Meatless burger, soy based	3 ounces
Meatless burger, vegetable and starch based	1
Nut spreads: almond butter, cashew butter, peanut butter, soy nut butter	1 tablespoon
Peas, cooked: black-eyed and split peas	½ cup
Refried beans, canned	½ cup
"Sausage" patties, soy based	1
Soy based "bacon" strips	3
Soy nuts, unsalted	¾ ounce
Tempeh	¼ cup
Tofu: regular, light	4 ounces (½ cup)

Nuts: An Important Caveat

The American Diabetes Association counts nuts as fats in small portions (see "The Fats List" in this chapter) but counts 1 tablespoon of nut butter as a protein even though it contains only $3\frac{1}{2}$ grams of protein (a standard protein choice has 7 grams of protein). Since nuts are about 700 to 800 calories per cup, practicing portion control when noshing on nuts is critical. With snacks, to reap the benefits without overdoing the calories, count $\frac{1}{2}$ ounce of nuts as a protein choice even though $\frac{1}{2}$ ounce averages only about 2 to 3 grams of protein. When $\frac{1}{2}$ ounce of nuts is eaten with a carb (like a fruit or handful of crackers) as part of a snack, both the protein and the fat lend a sense of fullness and satisfaction to the snack. For exactly what a half ounce of nuts looks like, see the chart in chapter 7 on page 120.

The Fats List

As discussed earlier, fats can be either good for you (in moderation) or bad for you. Healthy fats are monounsaturated fats (they help lower cholesterol and raise healthy HDL) and polyunsaturated fats (they help lower cholesterol). "Bad fats" are saturated fats (they raise lousy LDL cholesterol and are solid at room temperature) and trans fats (they raise cholesterol levels and are mostly artificially produced as hydrogenated and partially hydrogenated fats).

Things to consider: A fat choice is based on a serving that has 5 grams of total fat. Fats and oils are mixtures of several different types of fat. The predominant fat dictates which list it's in. The goal is to replace saturated fats with healthy fats, not to add healthy fats without taking unhealthy fats away. All fats contain 9 calories per gram. Too many calories consumed that aren't burned off will cause weight gain regardless of the source. Because the number of fat servings depends on the calories, there's no simple rule for the daily number of fat choices. For most people, a reasonable amount is 1 to 2 servings per meal. When choosing a spread, liquid vegetable oil should be the first ingredient in regular tub spread and the second ingredient after water in light spreads. All spreads should be trans fat–free. A tablespoon is about the size of your thumb, and a teaspoon is about the size of your thumb tip.

The Fats List

FOOD	SERVING SIZE
MONOUNSATURATED FATS	
Avocado, medium	2 tablespoons
Nut butters: almond, cashew, peanut	1½ teaspoons
Nuts	
Almonds	6
Brazil	2
Cashews	6
Hazelnuts	5
Macadamia	3
Mixed	6
Peanuts	10
Pecans	4 halves
Pistachios	16
Oil: canola, olive, peanut	1 teaspoon
Olives	
Black	8 large
Green	10 large
POLYUNSATURATED FATS	
Margarine: lower fat, trans fat–free	1 tablespoon
Margarine: tub or stick, trans fat–free	1 teaspoon
Mayonnaise	
Reduced fat	1 tablespoon
Regular	1 teaspoon
Mayonnaise-style salad dressing	
Reduced fat	1 tablespoon
Regular	2 teaspoons
Nuts	
Pine nuts	1 tablespoon
Walnuts	4 halves
Oil: corn, cottonseed, flaxseed, grape seed, safflower, soybean, sunflower	1 teaspoon
Plant stanol spreads (Benecol)	
Light	1 tablespoon
Regular	2 teaspoons

The Fats List, continued

FOOD	SERVING SIZE
Salad dressing (fat-free is on the Sweets list)	
Reduced fat	2 tablespoons
Regular	1 tablespoon
Seeds	
Flaxseed, whole	1 tablespoon
Pumpkin, sunflower	1 tablespoon
Sesame seeds	1 tablespoon
Tahini or sesame paste	2 teaspoons
SATURATED FATS	
Bacon, cooked, regular or turkey	1 slice (in larger portion is a fatty meat)
Butter	
Reduced fat	1 tablespoon
Stick	1 teaspoon
Whipped	2 teaspoons
Coconut, sweetened, shredded	2 tablespoons
Coconut milk	
Light	⅓ cup
Regular	1½ tablespoons
Cream	
Half-and-half	2 tablespoons
Heavy	1 tablespoon
Light	1½ tablespoons
Whipped	2 tablespoons
Whipped, pressurized	¼ cup
Cream cheese	
Reduced fat	1½ tablespoons
Regular	1 tablespoon
Lard	1 teaspoon
Oil: coconut, palm, palm kernel	1 teaspoon
Salt pork	¼ ounce
Shortening, solid	1 teaspoon
Sour cream	
Reduced fat or light	3 tablespoons
Regular	2 tablespoons

The Free Foods List

These foods contain fewer than 20 calories and 5 grams of carb in the serving size shown. Eaten in this amount, these foods are considered "free." In larger portions, however, they may start to add up to the point where you need to count them in your daily carb budget or factor in their calories. Other ingredients not to worry about: flavoring extracts, garlic, herbs, spices, nonstick cooking spray, hot pepper sauce, cooking wine, and Worcestershire sauce. Beware seasonings that contain salt. Many people with prediabetes are at risk for or have high blood pressure, which can be aggravated by eating too much sodium.

The Free Foods List

FOOD	SERVING SIZE
Barbecue sauce	2 teaspoons
Candy, hard (regular or sugar-free)	1 piece
Cream cheese, fat-free	1 tablespoon
Creamers	
Nondairy, liquid	1 tablespoon
Nondairy, powdered	2 teaspoons
Gelatin, sugar-free	unlimited
Gum (preferably sugar-free)	unlimited
Honey mustard	1 tablespoon
Horseradish	unlimited
Jam or jelly, light or no added sugar	2 teaspoons
Ketchup	1 tablespoon
Lemon juice	unlimited
Margarine spread	
Fat-free	1 tablespoon
Reduced fat	1 teaspoon
Miso	1½ teaspoons
Mustard	unlimited
Parmesan cheese, grated	1 tablespoon
Pickles	
Dill	1½ medium
Sweet, bread-and-butter	2 slices
Sweet, gherkin	¾ ounce

The Free Foods List, continued

FOOD	SERVING SIZE
Relish	1 tablespoon
Salad dressing	
Fat-free or low fat	1 tablespoon
Fat-free Italian	2 tablespoons
Salsa	¼ cup
Sour cream, fat-free or reduced fat	1 tablespoon
Soy sauce, light or regular	1 tablespoon
Sweet-and-sour sauce	2 teaspoons
Sweet chili sauce	2 teaspoons
Syrup, sugar-free	2 tablespoons
Taco sauce	1 tablespoon
Vinegar	unlimited
Whipped topping	
Light or fat-free	2 tablespoons
Regular	1 tablespoon
Yogurt, any type	2 tablespoons
DRINKS AND MIXES	
Carbonated water	any moderate amount
Club soda	any moderate amount
Cocoa powder, unsweetened	1 tablespoon
Coffee or tea, unsweetened or with sugar substitute	any moderate amount
Diet soft drinks	any moderate amount
Sugar-free drink mixes	any moderate amount
Tonic water, diet	any moderate amount
Water, flavored, carbohydrate-free	any moderate amount

This chapter has identified all the carbohydrate foods, categorized and portioned out into amounts that will deliver about 15 grams of carbohydrate into your bloodstream as glucose. Also outlined are foods that don't contain significant amounts of carbohydrates. As long as you make healthy choices, you can use these foods to fill up on without bumping up your blood sugar. Next in the prediabetes diet plan you'll learn how to mix and match carbohydrates with other noncarbohydrate-containing foods so that at meal or snack time you can continue to eat the foods you love without making your blood glucose levels surge. That brings us to the most important—and for many people the most challenging—part of eating healthier: meal planning. It takes time and energy, and often needs to be moved up your life list of important things to do. It is possible to be a mediocre cook and still eat healthfully. All you need is a little patience, a determination to budget out the time needed to make it happen, and a willingness to make some mistakes along the way.

Meal Planning on a Carb-Distributed Diet

So far we have been focused on what carbohydrates are, which foods contain them, and how they affect your blood glucose and insulin response. Now it's time to get down to where the rubber hits the road. How will meal planning help you manage your prediabetes? When planning a prediabetes-friendly meal, the first task is identifying which parts of the meal contain carbs (there may be more than one). For example, a dinner of chicken, corn, potato, and milk contains three carbohydrate foods—corn, potatoes (both starchy vegetables), and milk. A fruit or sweet dessert eaten after the meal will add more carbs. Switching out the corn for asparagus, carrots, or a salad will trim some carbs, leaving a few left in your budget for a small portion of dessert, if you like. This is a pretty simple example because each of the foods on the dinner plate are separate and they are easy to recognize on their own. Things get more complicated when carbs are wrapped up in other foods, in complex dishes that make them a combination of carbohydrates, protein, and fat. Carbs are harder to recognize in these combined foods.

Carbs and Combination Foods

Not all foods you eat are just a starch or a protein or a vegetable. Casseroles, stews, burritos, and pizza are made up of several food choices wrapped around each other. It is difficult but possible to count carbs in these circumstances. Use your best guess and assume there's probably a little more carbohydrate in the combination food than you think. The American Diabetes Association sells loads of meal-planning guides and cookbooks that break combination foods and recipes down into exchanges (see the ADA's website, www .diabetes.org). If the combination food or recipe provides a nutrient breakdown—many of them do nowadays—you can do the math yourself and figure out how many 15-gram "choices" are in a serving.

Let's look at a few examples of combination foods as listed in ADA's *Choose Your Foods: Exchange Lists for Diabetes.*[4] This should give you an idea of how you can break down just about any combination food:

- Burrito, 5 ounces (bean and beef) = three starches, one lean meat, and two fats
- Cheese pizza (one-quarter of a 12-inch pizza) = two starches and two medium-fat meats
- Chicken noodle soup, 1 cup = one carbohydrate
- Beef stew, 1 cup = one starch, one medium-fat meat, zero to three fats
- Macaroni salad, ½ cup = two starches and three fats

These exchange breakdowns are very specific, but what if you're standing in the aisle of the grocery store, package in hand, and you'd like to know how many carb choices are in a serving of a particular food? Simply look at the "Total Carbohydrate" line on the Nutrition Facts label and divide by 15 (the number of carb grams in one choice of a carb-containing food). For example:

- A veggie burger made mostly of vegetables and soy contains 13 grams of carbohydrate (4 of which is healthy indigestible dietary fiber), so it counts as approximately one choice. Enjoy the veggie burger surrounded by a standard store-bought, 150-calorie whole wheat hamburger bun, at 26 grams of carbohydrate (containing another 4 grams of dietary fiber because it's made with whole wheat), and you've added roughly another two carb choices. Serve this with a salad and a carb-free beverage, and you're right on target for a three-carb-serving—or 45-gram carb—meal.

- One-third of a ten-inch frozen cheese pizza contains 42 grams of carbohydrate. That's roughly three choices. Add some veggies to the pizza before you pop it in the oven, and serve with a large salad with reduced-fat dressing to help fill you up, and you've got a carb-controlled meal.

- You're at a Subway sandwich shop and order a six-inch lower-fat tur-key sandwich. The nutrition information provided by Subway says there are 46 grams of carbohydrate, which means the six-inch sub is the equivalent of eating three slices of bread, or three carb choices. Sounds like a good choice as long as you avoid eating many other carbs with your meal, like chips and soda.

Of course you still need to consider the total calories for the meal if you're trying to lose weight. Now that we've introduced the idea of com-bining foods to make a meal, let's look at how to start making this happen when preparing meals at home.

Planning Dinner

Now that you have your lists of carb-containing foods and know your por-tion sizes, you can start using your carb budget to control the amount of carbs you eat at a meal or snack. Remember, the ultimate goal of the bal-anced plate and exchange list system is to help you better understand what a reasonable amount of carbohydrate intake is for someone with insu-lin resistance. But eating smaller portions of carbs and spreading them out over the day should also help you control your calories—as long as you don't compensate by eating excessive amounts of protein foods or too much added fat. The balanced-plate, carb-distributed approach is designed to provide that "balanced diet" that's good for your health in many ways: you'll get enough protein to meet your nutritional needs and fill you up; you'll have enough healthy fat to meet your needs for fat-soluble nutrients and to make your food taste good; and you'll get a lot of plant foods to increase your intake of fiber and health-promoting phytonutrients—these will also take up space on your plate and in your stomach so that it's easier to avoid eating too many grains (starches) and other carbs.

As tempting as it may be, be careful not to over-restrict carbs either. You'll then be practicing an unsustainable behavior, which may trigger reactive overeating later in the day due to low blood sugar. Start with a reasonably sized plate, which in your kitchen may be a ten-inch salad plate. In this example we'll use someone aiming for a goal of 45 grams of carbohydrate for dinner. Let's begin with protein. For women, serve a 3- to 4-ounce portion of protein to cover roughly 25 percent of the plate. Men, or more physically active women, may need more protein, maybe 4 to 6 ounces. Remember, all these suggestions are averages. To learn more specifically what *your* allowance is, consider meeting with a registered dietitian for an individualized consultation.

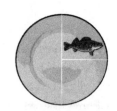
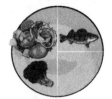
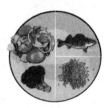

Now cover half the plate with nonstarchy vegetables. This can be a large portion of a cooked vegetable,

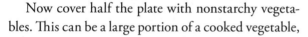

Bread: Mind the Two Qs

We all love bread in one form or another, but it's easy to eat too much. Choosing bread is a classic example of where the Two Qs can steer you in the right direction. It's about the quality (choosing whole grain breads, rolls, bagels, English muffins, and tortillas over white flour options) and the quantity (you have to include them in your carb budget). As a general rule, I suggest avoiding bread with meals unless it *is* the carb, as in a sandwich with lunch, a whole wheat English muffin with breakfast, or one slice toasted with reduced-fat cheese or a thin layer of peanut butter for a snack. What you want to avoid is already having a carb choice planned for the meal and then eating bread on top of that (like that tempting never-ending bread basket in restaurants).

One way to enjoy bread without guilt is to have it as the starch choice at dinner. In our house we love good-quality bread, so occasionally we'll have a hearty, protein-dense salad and eat bread as the starch. It's bread *as* the carb—no reason not to enjoy it. When reading bread labels, look for three things: the first ingredient should include the word "whole," as in whole wheat or whole oat; the fiber should be 2 to 3 grams per slice; and the calories should be in the 60- to 90-calorie range. Calories matter, and a slice of bread should weigh roughly 1 ounce (30 grams by weight). Some breads list that prized 2 to 3 grams of fiber, but at a cost of 110 to 150 calories per slice.

a large salad containing several different vegetables, or one portion of a cooked vegetable and a small salad.

Next let's calculate the carbohydrate piece, starting with the starch. If you look back at the starch list, one option is ⅓ cup of cooked brown rice, which is 15 grams of carbohydrate or one carb choice. Sounds tiny, I know. But when you pack cooked rice into a measuring cup—which you need to do to actually see what ⅓ cup cooked rice looks like—and then dump it on your plate, it may seem bigger. You have at a minimum 45 grams of carbohydrate to work with, so depending on what other carbs you eat at that meal, you may be able to eat two portions of rice (⅔ cup)—or 30 grams of carbs. For this example, let's assume you're going with one serving of rice, which populates the remaining quarter of the plate.

You've now used up 15 grams of your 45-gram carb budget (one of your three choices for the meal), leaving you with 30 grams to "spend" during the rest of your meal (if you have a 60-gram carb budget, you can go for that two servings of brown rice and still be left with 30 grams of carbs). If you add an 8-ounce glass of 1 percent milk (one carb choice) and a cup of cubed cantaloupe (one carb choice), you've now hit your budget of roughly 45 grams of carbohydrate for the meal.

If you've already eaten your recommended minimum of two fruits this day, you may decide to spend 15 grams of carbohydrate on a dessert instead of a fruit, maybe ½ cup of sugar-free ice cream. This is how you work in your special treats. You make room for them in your diet by making smart decisions throughout the day. Limit how often you decide to spend a chunk of your carb budget on foods without any nutritional value, however. Much of the benefit from eating more healthfully is the positive feeling you get when you fill up on good-quality food, which is unlikely to happen with too much processed food, even if it doesn't deliver a lot of carbs.

Let's look at some other examples of carb-controlled meals using 45 grams and 60 grams of carbs per meal as the goal. People who are allowed more carbs can add them accordingly.

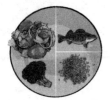

Carb-Controlled Meals

45-GRAM CARB BUDGET	60-GRAM CARB BUDGET
3–4 ounces grilled chicken	3–4 ounces grilled chicken
½ cup mashed potato (1 choice)	1 cup mashed potato (2 choices)
1 cup broccoli	1 cup broccoli
Salad with 1–2 tablespoons low-fat dressing	Salad with 1–2 tablespoons low-fat dressing
8 ounces 1 percent milk (1 choice)	8 ounces skim milk (1 choice)
1 medium orange (1 choice)	1¼ cups sliced strawberries (1 choice)

Either of these meals could be adjusted by using the exchange lists to make alternative choices. Here are some different ideas:

- In either of these meals, the 3- to 4-ounce portion of chicken could be swapped out for a same-size portion of turkey, fish, lean meat, tofu, or other protein choice.
- The starch choice can be swapped out for any other serving of starch from the starch list. Your trade-off could be brown rice, couscous, pasta (preferably whole wheat or at least one of the pasta blends with added protein), sweet potato, winter squash, corn, peas—your choice.
- The vegetables are nonstarchy, so we don't count their carbs toward our daily carb budget. Any vegetable or salad listed as nonstarchy in the exchange lists is considered a "freebie" unless it's fried or loaded with butter, cream, or cheese sauce.
- The carb content of milk doesn't change with the fat content, so either skim or 1 percent is a healthy choice. Two percent milk is very close to whole milk, which is about 3.25 percent milk fat, so those who like thicker milk should opt for one of the enhanced creamier-tasting low-fat or fat-free milks.
- The fruit choice could be any of the fresh, canned, or dried options in the fruit list. Juice should be limited to around ⅓ to ½ cup per day, otherwise it's best to opt for whole fruit choices. Juice is a lot easier to go overboard on. One medium-sized fresh fruit has the same calories as only about ½ cup of fruit juice, which contains no fiber and doesn't contribute to a feeling of fullness the way whole fruit does.

- You could make the 60-gram carb meal a 75-gram carb meal by increasing the potatoes to 1½ cups or mixing 6 ounces of light yogurt in with your strawberries.

Planning Lunch

The meal may be different, but the same rules apply. The examples below consist of one sandwich meal and one salad-based lunch.

The 60-gram carb meal could be increased to 75 grams of carb by adding 8 ounces of 1 percent milk or a cup of broth-based soup. As with dinner, you can mix it up by changing your choices. Here are some creative ideas:

- The turkey for the sandwich could be replaced with tuna (with low-fat mayonnaise), ham, lean roast beef, canned chicken, or hummus and avocado.
- The chicken in the salad could be replaced with leftover salmon, tuna, boiled eggs, grated reduced-fat cheese, and beans.
- The pita could be replaced with a slice or two of whole grain bread. Two slices of light wheat bread (two slices of reduced-calorie bread is one choice) could be used to make a whole sandwich for the 45-gram carb plan.
- For the 60-gram plan, half the pita could be replaced with 1 cup of broth-based soup, which counts as one starch.
- The lettuce and tomato on the sandwich and the carrots on the side could be replaced with a salad.
- Eight ounces of skim or 1 percent milk could substitute for the light yogurt.

Lunch: Sandwich or Salad?

45-GRAM CARB BUDGET	60-GRAM CARB BUDGET
3 ounces turkey or 2 ounces turkey and 1 ounce cheese	3 ounces grilled chicken
Mustard or low-fat mayonnaise	Low-fat salad dressing
Half a 6-inch whole wheat pita (1 choice)	6-inch whole wheat pita (2 choices)
Lettuce and tomato	Lettuce, tomato, cucumber, peppers, onions
Baby carrots dipped in low-fat dressing	Carrots, mushrooms, and so on
12 cherries (1 choice)	⅓ cantaloupe (1 choice)
6 ounces light yogurt (1 choice)	6 ounces light yogurt (1 choice)

Planning Breakfast

Breakfasts are often carb heavy and fairly low in protein. Adding a protein source helps you feel fuller for longer, maybe allowing you to make it to lunch without snacking.

There are many ways to mix up breakfast. Here are some different ideas for keeping it interesting:

- The ½ cup of oatmeal can be replaced with ¾ cup of unsweetened dry cereal.
- The ½ banana and ½ serving of milk can be replaced with a whole banana; it's fine to still put a dash of milk in your oatmeal.
- One tablespoon of sugar, brown sugar, or honey is one carb choice, so if you want to add a teaspoon or two of sweetener to your oatmeal, just be sure to watch the carbs from other sources.
- The ½ to 1 whole banana can be replaced with 1 to 2 tablespoons of raisins or another dried fruit in your oatmeal or dry cereal. Add a tablespoon of chopped nuts to add a little more protein and fiber to your cereal.
- The whole wheat English muffin can be replaced with two slices of whole grain toast, a small (approximately 150-calorie) bagel, two waffles, or two small (4-inch-diameter) pancakes.
- Two egg whites or a ¼ cup of egg substitutes could substitute for the whole egg.
- In a pinch, a PB&J with 1 to 2 tablespoons of peanut butter, a teaspoon or two of 100 percent fruit spread, and two slices of whole wheat bread can be a pretty filling breakfast on the run.

Breakfast Planning

45-GRAM CARB BUDGET	60-GRAM CARB BUDGET
½ cup cooked oatmeal (1 choice)	1 whole wheat English muffin (2 choices)
4 ounces 1 percent milk (½ choice)	1 egg, fried in nonstick spray
Half a banana (½ choice)	Half a large grapefruit (1 choice)
8 ounces 1 percent milk (1 choice)	2 teaspoons tub spread for muffin
Coffee or tea	Coffee or tea

Snacks That Satisfy

When planning snacks, pairing a carb with protein will make the snack more satisfying and slow the delivery of glucose into your blood. Use the exchange lists to plan snacks the same way: one carb choice (or two if your budget allows for 30 grams of carb at a snack) and one protein serving. If you opt for leaner protein choices—or small portions of higher-fat choices—you'll save some calories. Here are some examples of snacks that pair one carb choice with one lean protein:

- 5 whole wheat crackers and 1 ounce reduced-fat cheese
- 1 apple and 1 ounce reduced-fat cheese
- Half of a 6-inch pita with 1 ounce of turkey (with a touch of mustard or salsa for added flavor)

It's possible to opt for a higher-fat snack, but it's important to really watch your portions to control calories:

- 5 whole wheat crackers with 1 tablespoon peanut butter
- 1 egg and 1 slice whole wheat toast with 1 teaspoon of tub spread

Nuts contain a small amount of protein when eaten in small amounts, which is absolutely necessary if you don't want nuts to be a major calorie contributor to your diet. Mindlessly noshing on ½ cup of peanuts will load you down with 425 calories and 36 grams of fat, but a few nuts combined with a carb can make for a satisfying snack. Try these combos:

- 17 grapes and 10 to 15 peanuts
- ¾ cup unsweetened cereal (or ¼ cup granola) and 6 to 10 almonds
- 6 ounces light yogurt and 1 tablespoon chopped walnuts

More snack ideas are available in chapter 7.

Counting Carbs Using Food Labels

Up to this point we've mostly been talking about using the exchange lists to estimate the carbohydrate content of foods. But you can also use the food labels that appear on the packaging (see the example opposite). All the information is there: the serving size, the grams of carbohydrate per serving, and the grams of fiber (if it's 5 grams or more of fiber, you can subtract half from the total carbs). If the grams of fiber aren't an even number, round up. The accuracy of your carb count is only as good as you are at judging the portion size. Let's look at an example of estimating an appropriate portion of cereal for someone aiming for two carb choices (30 grams of carb) of cereal for breakfast:

Fiber Flakes

Serving size: ¾ cup

Total carbohydrate: 23 grams

Fiber: 5 grams

Because the fiber is 5 grams or more, you can subtract half the fiber from the carb total, so there are roughly 20 grams of absorbable carbohydrates in the ¾ cup serving (23 grams of total carbohydrate minus half the fiber rounded up to 3 grams). If you divide 20 into 30, you get 1.5 servings, or slightly more than 1 cup of cereal (0.75 cup × 1.5 = 1.125 cups). If you have an aversion to doing math, don't sweat it. Estimate. Guess. At least you're making an effort to think about the portion. Measure the portion out a few times so you become a pretty good estimator. You'll need to learn this skill to do a quick check of whether a food in the grocery store is a good choice. If you add a glass of milk and a fruit to your portion of cereal (two choices, or 30 grams of carb), you arrive at about 60 grams of carbohydrate for that meal. Aiming for 45 grams? Stick with one serving of cereal or have half a fruit serving (for example, half a small banana instead of a whole one) and half of a milk serving (4 ounces instead of 8 ounces). A warning about labels: Don't expect the manufacturer's portion size to be the same as the exchange list. Many store-bought breads, for example, weigh more than 1 ounce, so they are more than 15 grams of carb per slice.

Reality Check on Portion Sizes

All the portions in these examples come from the American Diabetes Association's exchange lists and are designed to help you see what reasonable portion really look like. When you compare them to what many of us are accustomed to eating, it becomes clear how dramatically portion sizes have increased over the years—in some instances more than twice the size they used to be! Having said that, I don't feel there is a significant difference between eating half an ounce or three-quarters of an ounce of crackers. Or between a 4-ounce or 5-ounce apple. Those aren't the kinds of portion control errors we're making that have made the United States one of the most overweight nations in the world. Our challenges are more on the scale of portions that are 50 to 100 percent bigger than they should be. We're talking several hundred too many calories, not just the few calories' difference between six and eight crackers.

As you lament portion sizes perhaps a bit smaller than what you're used to, keep in mind that depending on your carb budget, you may be able to eat two servings (two choices) of one carb-containing food at a time. You may decide to spend two of your three or four carb choices at a meal on one thing, like ⅔ cup of brown rice or pasta instead of ⅓ cup. You just need to make room for it within your per meal carb-distribution budget. It's important to accept there's a certain amount of discomfort that goes along with eating less, mainly because what we're often presented with—particularly in restaurants and takeout containers—is excessive, requiring us to resist some of the food we're exposed to. It is possible to adjust to eating smaller portions over time. Many others have done it, and so can you.

Basic Principles

Carb counting is one way to help you relearn reasonable portion sizes of carb-containing foods. As you start to practice eating more appropriate portions, there are a few simple prediabetes diet plan rules you can apply to healthfully distribute your carbs over the day.

Fruit. Whole fruits should be limited to one serving at a time, using the fruit exchange list as a way to estimate a portion. Juice should be limited to no more than 4 to 6 ounces a day. To get your minimum of two fruits a day, have one either with breakfast or a midmorning snack and one in the afternoon or evening.

Milk or yogurt. Eat these one serving at a time. If you're having milk with breakfast, have yogurt as a snack in the afternoon.

Grains and starchy vegetables. Limit these to two servings per meal or one serving per snack (possibly more if you're tall, male, or very physically active). At least half of your grains should be whole grains.

Sweets. Don't just add them to your diet; be sure to budget them in. Look at the food label on the packaging and see how many 15-gram carb units a portion of the food will gobble up. If a label isn't available (say, you're enjoying a home-baked treat), assume that our usual instinct is to eat larger portions than we should, so keep it small. A word to the wise: Think twice before keeping a stash of sweets in your house. Can you really limit it to just one small portion a day? Maybe you know yourself very well and you can do this, but most people find it hard to resist reaching into the cookie jar. It's possible to budget a little something sweet into your day, but usually there are enough of these special treats floating around our food environment without stocking your cupboards with things that will present a constant source of temptation!

7

Making It Happen: Meals and Snacks

You've committed to managing your prediabetes by following the pre-diabetes diet plan. Whether you choose the balanced-plate approach or the more structured carb-counting approach, your desired outcome is that most days you'll eat pretty well. Now you need to set the stage for that to happen. If you want to eat well, you have to have good food choices close at hand. You need to make time to prepare your meals and snacks, and time to pack up your food if it's leaving the house with you in the morning. To have good food choices available, you need to carve out time each week to go to the grocery store (I encourage you to share this responsibility with a spouse or partner!). To have the time to shop, you need to plan for it as you would anything else you deem important. This "planning" part eludes many would-be healthier eaters. But if you're trying to avoid diabetes, you have to prioritize this as the most important thing in your life right now.

If you don't take time to think about your next meal before you're starving, the chances of grabbing something not so good is high. That doesn't mean you have to cook elaborate meals from scratch every night. I'm all for shortcuts as long as they result in reasonable choices. But you do need to put at least *some* effort into planning and preparing meals. With fewer people cooking these days, knowledge of how to plan and cook meals is falling by the wayside, leaving increasing numbers of people eating out more and gaining weight. Let's walk through the day—meal by meal—and review some simple suggestions to help make meal planning go a little smoother.

Begin with Breakfast

Let's start with some breakfast rules:

1. The number-one rule, if you want to control your insulin resistance and lose weight, is that you have to eat breakfast. There is no way around it.

2. If the food or combination food is a healthy choice and stays within your carb budget for the meal, it's an option. Your breakfast could be as simple as peanut butter and fruit spread on whole wheat bread. You choose what works for the prediabetes diet plan and for you.

3. Make sure you budget ten to fifteen minutes into your morning, either at home or at work, to eat breakfast. Ideally you'll be eating mindfully (without distractions), but in the end what matters most is that you do eat breakfast.

4. Accept that a breakfast you eat at home or bring to work is probably more healthy than the pastries or giant-sized muffins you'll get at the coffee shop or be offered at a breakfast meeting.

So what are the usual mistakes people make?

- Skipping breakfast—by far the most common mistake. Studies show that people who skip breakfast tend to eat more at night, which can be a potential contributor to weight gain.

- Thinking that coffee with cream and sugar or artificial sweetener is breakfast. It's not! It certainly doesn't add the valuable nutrients your body needs to kick off your day and jump-start your metabolism.

- Grabbing breakfast where you get your morning coffee (unless that favorite morning spot is your own kitchen and you're preparing your own breakfast). Even if you find what appears to be a healthy choice at the corner café, the portion size is often enormous. If you have time to wait in line at a coffee shop, you can probably find ten minutes to grab a quick bowl of cereal or a whole wheat English muffin with peanut butter at home before leaving the house.

If you're a regular breakfast skipper, start by believing you have the power to change this habit. Of course you're busy in the morning, and it's not easy to change morning routines. Be patient and give yourself a chance to establish a new habit. This one really matters. Start by budgeting in a few extra minutes in the morning. Keep it simple by grabbing a piece of fruit or a yogurt. Next you can work on making a more balanced choice.

Carb-Friendly Breakfasts

Assuming you're working with a 45- to 75-gram carb budget for the breakfast meal and want to include a protein source, you've got a lot of options. You may opt for a slightly smaller 30 gram carb breakfast (maybe by replacing a carb-containing beverage for one that's carb-free), but you want to make sure you get in enough carbs at breakfast time to keep your blood glucose levels in a stable range until your midmorning snack or lunch. Don't like traditional breakfast foods? The chart that follows includes some unconventional options, too.

Healthy Breakfast Options

BREAKFAST CHOICE	CARBS (GRAMS)	
One whole wheat English muffin	30	
1 tablespoon peanut or other nut butter	0	**45 grams total**
8 ounces 1 percent or skim milk	15	
Two slices whole wheat toast (15 grams each)	30	
½ cup 1 percent or nonfat cottage cheese	0	
8 ounces 1 percent or skim milk	15	**60 grams total**
One-third cantaloupe	15	
One whole wheat English muffin	30	
One egg or one serving egg substitute (combined with English muffin as an egg sandwich)	0	
1 tablespoon tub spread	0	**45 grams total**
8 ounces 1 percent or skim milk	15	
2 whole wheat waffles	30	
1 tablespoon peanut or other nut butter	0	
One small banana	15	**60 grams total**
8 ounces 1 percent or skim milk	15	
One (six-inch) whole wheat tortilla	15	
One egg scrambled and cooked with nonstick spray and a slice of reduced-fat cheese	0	
One pear	15	**45 grams total**
8 ounces 1 percent or skim milk	15	

Healthy Breakfast Options, continued

BREAKFAST CHOICE	CARBS (GRAMS)	
1 cup cooked old-fashioned or steel-cut oatmeal	30	**45 grams total**
1 tablespoon chopped walnuts	0	
2 tablespoons dried cranberries or raisins	15	
1 cup shredded wheat cereal	30	**75 grams total**
¾ cup blueberries	15	
1 tablespoon chopped nuts	0	
8 ounces 1 percent or skim milk	15	
1 slice whole wheat toast with tub spread	15	
6 ounces plain, artificially sweetened, or Greek yogurt	15	**60 grams total**
2 tablespoons dried fruit	15	
¼ cup low-fat granola	15	
1 tablespoon chopped nuts	0	
Half cup canned pineapple (in water)	15	
Two slices whole grain bread	30	**60 grams total**
Two slices reduced-fat cheese (melted on top of the bread)	0	
One apple	15	
8 ounces 1 percent milk	15	
One (six-inch) whole wheat tortilla	15	**40–42 grams total**
2 ounces leftover chicken	0	
17 grapes (roughly a fistful)	15	
6 ounces sugar-free hot chocolate	10–12 grams (check the food label)	
Ten Ak-Mak stone ground sesame crackers	40 (2 servings per the food label)	**55 grams total**
Two Laughing Cow spreadable cheese wedges	0	
4 ounces orange juice	15	
1 ounce (30 grams) whole grain crackers	15–20 (the number of crackers varies by type—check the food label)	**45–50 grams total**
⅓ cup hummus	15	
One small orange	15	

Healthy Breakfast Options, continued

BREAKFAST CHOICE	CARBS (GRAMS)	
One small bagel (such as Original Lender's frozen) or bagel thin	30	
One slice turkey	0	
One slice cheese	0	**45 grams total**
1 teaspoon light mayonnaise or mustard	0	
Lettuce and tomato	0	
8 ounces 1 percent or skim milk	15	

Any of these breakfast suggestions could be trimmed by 15 grams of carb by transporting some of the breakfast carbs to a midmorning snack. Another option for those who prefer a smaller breakfast is to have half of your breakfast first thing in the morning and half as a midmorning snack. Or it could be two-thirds at breakfast and one-third midmorning. Experiment and see what works best for you.

Midmorning Snack, or Not?

If you're aiming to control your insulin resistance, is a midmorning snack necessary? That depends on how filling your breakfast was and how hungry you'll be by lunchtime if you don't snack. One way to enhance the odds of making it to lunch without needing a snack is to eat more protein. Adding eggs, low-fat cottage cheese, or Greek yogurt (which is higher in protein than regular yogurt) to your breakfast may help you feel fuller longer—and therefore less in need of a snack before lunch. Studies have shown old-fashioned oatmeal (not the flavored kind with tons of added sugar!) to be super-satisfying, keeping hunger at bay for a longer period of time.

If you do feel you need a midmorning snack, try limiting it to a piece of fruit if possible, because breakfast and lunch are generally much closer together than lunch and dinner. Most people don't eat enough fruit, so checking off one fruit serving midmorning fulfills half of your two-a-day minimum requirement by lunch. Keeping this snack smaller will also help you save calories in the morning that may be better spent on an afternoon snack, when something more substantial may be needed to help control your hunger before dinner. If you do need a little protein, keep it small, such as a tablespoon of nut butter on a few crackers or six to eight almonds with a fruit.

Let's Do Lunch!

As for your midday meal, the prediabetes diet plan has some important rules:

1. The number-one lunchtime rule: don't skip it! Skipping lunch can be a setup for reactive overeating that begins in front of the vending machine at 4 p.m. and doesn't stop until bedtime. As I've mentioned before, eating patterns matter. Even if lunch starts as a half-lunch grabbed at your desk before a meeting, do it! You can always finish it later, and it's better than waiting to eat anything until later when you're starved and out of control.

2. Consider flipping lunch and dinner so lunch is the larger meal. It may help you control your hunger better for the rest of the day. According to a recent study published in the *International Journal of Obesity*, eating your main meal earlier in the day may offer weight-loss advantages as well. In this study of more than four hundred people in Spain, where lunch is the main meal of the day, those who ate their main meal before 3 p.m. lost significantly more weight on a similar number of calories.[1] Until recent times, lunch was "dinner" for many in this country as well—and people were a lot thinner!

3. Some people do better splitting lunch in two, eating half at noon and the other half at 3 or 4 p.m. This basically means eating a meal or minimeal every four hours or so, which may help you stay ahead of your hunger as the day rolls on.

4. Find a way to work both fruits and vegetables into your lunch. You'll walk away feeling a lot fuller on fewer calories and won't feel pressured to fit all your fruits and vegetables for the day into dinner.

5. If you can't pack a lunch from home, check out all your employee cafeteria offerings to see if you can piece together a decent lunch à la carte. A nice salad-bar salad with a variety of colorful vegetables, two to three options of added protein (grilled chicken, half a hard-boiled egg, and a small sprinkling of grated or crumbled cheese works nicely), and a tablespoon of raisins or dried cranberries, topped with half a dressing ladle of low-cal dressing makes for a calorie-controlled but satisfying lunch. Or order the meat, chicken,

or fish option (watch the creamy sauces) with two side vegetables. In general, it's preferable to avoid the grill area unless it's to grab a piece of grilled chicken.

6. If you're bringing lunch from home, try to make it the night before while you're cleaning the kitchen and not yet settled in for the night. Waiting until morning to make your lunch increases the odds you'll get busy and forget.

What are the usual mistakes people make with their midday meal? You may see yourself making a few of these:

- Skipping lunch altogether. Just don't do it!
- Getting busy with work and eating lunch too late, at which point you'll probably be overhungry and at high risk for eating too much of the wrong thing when you finally get around to eating.
- Eating too little to hold you over for a decent amount of time. A salad with too little protein, fat-free dressing, and pita bread will not fill the void in your stomach for long.
- Going into business lunches starving and at high risk for grabbing a huge sandwich, a bag of chips, and a Frisbee-sized cookie—a carb-overload disaster for people with prediabetes.
- Being unrealistic about the challenges of eating healthfully in a restaurant. Assume that if you eat out, you're probably going to be served at least 25 to 30 percent more food than you should be eating. Sandwiches are often huge and served with fries, and there's often a lot more hidden fat in restaurant meals than you realize. This doesn't mean you can't enjoy the occasional dining-out lunch experience, but be a realist here. If you want to develop a healthy lifestyle, you have to come up with alternatives to the regular eating out many of us have become so accustomed to.

Lunch Menu Ideas

As with breakfast, under the prediabetes diet plan, aim for a 45- to 75-gram carb budget for lunch. Because lunch and dinner are fairly far apart for most people, including a 3- to 4-ounce portion of protein with lunch will slow digestion, helping to steady your blood glucose levels and keep you feeling fuller longer. Think of vegetables first, not last (remember the balanced-plate approach). Vegetables can be raw in the form of a salad, carrots, or sliced peppers or celery (or any other vegetable you like raw); cooked as a broth-based vegetable soup; or leftover reheated vegetables from last night's dinner. Fruit can be a piece of whole fruit, a serving of fruit salad, or a couple of tablespoons of dried fruit sprinkled into a salad. Watch those added fats—difficult to do if you're eating out often. The usual offenders are mayonnaise (100 calories per tablespoon); too much full-fat salad dressing (can be 80 to 180 calories per 2-tablespoon serving); too much cheese; sandwiches grilled in too much butter; cream soups; and everybody's favorite vice, fries.

Throughout the list of lunch options offered below, I'll point out free and combination foods from the exchange lists so you can see why some foods that have small amounts of carb are counted as free and other less obvious choices count either all or in part as a carb (like broth-based soup, for example). Nonstarchy vegetables are considered freebies, so we count their carbs as zero. We're working with estimates here. Don't sweat the small stuff.

Healthy Lunch Options

LUNCH CHOICE	CARBS (GRAMS)	
Two slices whole wheat bread (15 grams per slice)	30	
Two slices turkey, one slice cheese	0	
2 teaspoons low-fat mayonnaise or 1 tablespoon avocado	0	**60 grams total**
Lettuce and tomato	0	
8 ounces 1 percent or skim milk	15	
17 grapes (a handful)	15	
Half (six-inch) whole wheat pita	15	
2 ounces lean roast beef, one slice cheese	0	**45 grams total**
2 teaspoons barbecue sauce*	0	*(*Up to this amount is free on the exchange list.)*
Romaine lettuce, sliced red peppers	0	
One pear	15	
8 ounces skim or 1 percent milk	15	
One slice whole wheat bread	15	
1 tablespoon peanut butter	0	
1 teaspoon 100 percent fruit spread**	0	**45 grams total**
1 cup chicken noodle soup*	15	** = 1 carb "combination food"*
1 cup baby carrots and chopped celery	0	*** = Negligible amount of carbs.*
2 tablespoons low-fat dressing for dipping**	0	
One apple	15	
Lettuce, tomato, cucumbers, onions, peppers, and so on	0	
3 ounces grilled chicken	0	
½ cup kidney or garbanzo beans	15	**45 grams total**
2 tablespoons low-fat dressing	0	
Half (six-inch) whole wheat pita	15	
One packet sugar-free instant hot chocolate	15	
One small hamburger or cheeseburger patty	0	
One small bun	30	**45 grams total**
1 tablespoon ketchup*	0	*(*Up to this amount is free on the exchange list.)*
Side salad with low-fat dressing	0	
8 ounces skim or 1 percent milk	15	

Healthy Lunch Options, continued

LUNCH CHOICE	CARBS (GRAMS)	
Two slices whole grain bread	30	**45 grams total**
Two slices cheese (melted on top of the bread)	0	
One slice tomato (on top of cheese)	0	
1 cup baby carrots	0	
½ cup fruit cocktail in juice or water	15	
Sugar-free beverage	0	
Half (12-inch) thin crust cheese pizza	60	**75 grams total**
Side salad with low-fat dressing	0	
One orange	15	
Water or sugar-free beverage	0	
2 cups bean soup (lentil, pea, black bean)	30	**75 grams total** *(Note: The bean soup also counts as protein.)*
One small roll	15	
Two small plums	15	
8 ounces 1 percent milk	15	
One small (six-inch) sub roll	30–45	**45–60 grams total**
3 ounces turkey, ham, or roast beef	0	
Lettuce, tomato, onions, peppers, pickles	0	
1–2 teaspoons mustard or low-fat mayo	0	
8 ounces skim or 1 percent milk	15	
¾ cup 1 percent cottage cheese (equals 3 ounces of protein)	0	**45 grams total**
1 ounce (30 grams) of whole grain crackers	15	
1 cup cubed cantaloupe	15	
Two small (2¼-inch) chocolate chip cookies	15	
Water or sugar-free beverage	0	
4 ounces chicken or fish	0	**60 grams total**
½ cup cooked carrots	0	
½ cup cooked green beans	0	
1 cup brown or white rice	45	
6 ounces light yogurt	15	
Water or sugar-free beverage	0	

Healthy Lunch Options, continued

LUNCH CHOICE	CARBS (GRAMS)	
One (six-inch) whole wheat tortilla	15	
¼ cup tabouli	(negligible carbs)	
½ cup black beans	15	
Roasted red pepper slices	0	**60 grams total**
⅓ cup shredded part-skim cheese	0	
One apple	15	
8 ounces skim or 1 percent milk	15	
2 tablespoons peanut butter	0	
1 ounce (30 grams) whole grain crackers	15	**45 grams total** *(Note: The added sugar per serving in the peanut butter is negligible.)*
1 cup tomato soup	15	
Carrot and celery sticks	0	
8 ounces skim or 1 percent milk	15	
One medium baked potato	30	
1 cup chili	30	
¼ cup shredded part-skim cheese	0	**60 grams total**
Side salad with low-fat dressing	0	
Water or sugar-free beverage	0	
3–4 ounces chicken or shrimp	0	
1 cup stir-fried vegetables	0	
⅔ cup brown rice or white rice	30	**75 grams total**
One egg roll (half if eaten with duck sauce)	30	
½ cup pineapple chunks	15	

Reasonable Salads

Salads are an awesome filler, helping you feel like you've eaten a lot while actually consuming very few calories. But this assumes you stick with mostly vegetable-only ingredients. Fat-laden add-ons have the potential to really crank up the calories. Avoid altogether (or use very little of) the following: croutons, bacon bits, pasta salad, potato salad, large amounts of cheese, and oil-based bean salad mixes. Healthy fat choices worthy of a small sprinkle on your salad (roughly a teaspoon or two) include nuts, seeds, olives, and soy nuts. To ensure that your salad will really fill you up, aim for at least five ingredients, including at least four vegetables and a sprinkling of some sort of protein (beans, nuts, eggs, or reduced-fat cheese). Try adding a teaspoon or two of dried cranberries or raisins for added nutrients and texture. Aim for a rainbow of color: deep green lettuce, red tomatoes, yellow peppers, black olives, orange carrots, and light green cucumbers.

Most important, don't drown your salad in dressing! The universal portion is two tablespoons. Measure it out. Compare the calories—some full-fat varieties contain over 200 calories in two tablespoons, whereas low-fat varieties can have far fewer calories. I'm a fan of smaller amounts of low-fat salad dressing versus larger amounts of fat-free, as low-fat versions tend to taste better and the fat in the dressing helps us absorb many of the fat-soluble phytonutrients found in plant foods. Opt for heart-healthy olive oil or canola oil whenever possible, which can count for your small amount of healthful fat included in your meal. Not a big fan of bottled dressings? Make your own or use dry salad dressing packets that come with the glass bottle where you choose your source of vinegar and oil (use a little of both olive and canola and the fat won't solidify in the fridge). You simply follow the directions on the packets for "less oil" dressing.

Midafternoon Snack

Many people who struggle with portion control need something to fill the void during that long stretch between lunch and dinner, particularly because dinnertime is a lot later than it used to be. Incorporating an afternoon snack into your carb-distributed diet plan helps keep hunger under control to help you avoid overeating at dinner. The key is to plan for a balanced (part-carb, part-protein) snack that includes a portion of carbohydrate to keep your blood glucose levels from dipping and triggering carb cravings and a portion of lean protein to steady glucose levels and help you feel full.

Eating Nuts Without Going Nuts

Despite their fat content, in small amounts nuts can be an important part of a healthy diet. Yes, they are 80 percent fat, but they are also a good source of fiber, plant protein, healthful monounsaturated fat, vitamins, and minerals. With nuts, portion control is key. Instead of mindlessly noshing on nuts in front of the TV, try incorporating a handful into foods: sprinkle them on cereals or salads, mix them into a homemade trail mix, or stir them into yogurt. To avoid calorie overload, limit nuts to $\frac{1}{2}$-ounce portions and pair them with a carb, such as a fruit or light yogurt, for a filling snack. Ever wondered what $\frac{1}{2}$-ounce portions of your favorite nuts look like? See the chart on this page to learn the appropriate serving size.

Peanut butter and other nut butters can be healthy additions in the prediabetes diet plan as long as you're mindful of portions. Nut butters average around 100 calories per tablespoon. If there was ever a food to measure, this is it.

Nut Portion Sizes and Calories

NUT	NUTS PER ½ OUNCE	CALORIES PER ½ OUNCE
Almonds	11	85
Brazil nuts	3–4	93
Cashews	9	81
Hazelnuts	10	89
Macadamia nuts	5–6	102
Peanuts	14	83
Pecans	10	100
Pine nuts	1½ tablespoons	72
Pistachio nuts	23	81
Walnuts	7 halves	93

The Truth About Crackers

Serving sizes on cracker boxes vary considerably depending on how many crackers weigh an ounce (30 grams), the standard portion size for crackers and many other foods. Because crackers on their own aren't very filling, and eating them alone can easily escalate into eating too many, I recommend pairing a half a serving (½ ounce) of crackers with a protein, like reduced-fat cheese, tuna mixed with light mayo, 1 percent cottage cheese, or a small amount of peanut butter, bean dip, or hummus. In general, a ½-ounce serving of crackers is about 10 grams of carb, which is close enough to the 15-gram carb portions to consider it a carb choice. See the shopping list on page 178 for my recommended healthy cracker options.

Snack Suggestions

Being prepared—for almost every meal and snack—is an important part of establishing healthy eating habits. To make this easier, load up on snack baggies (half-size storage bags); small plastic containers for things like hummus, peanut butter, and low-fat salad dressings; and an insulated lunch bag and ice pack to carry it all to work. Try these easy and delicious snack ideas, or use them as a blueprint for a snack you'll find satisfying:

- ½ cup 1 percent cottage cheese and ½ cup canned fruit in water or juice
- ½ cup cottage cheese flavored with herb seasoning and ½ ounce of crackers and/or vegetables
- ½ cup tuna mixed with light mayo and ½ ounce of crackers
- 1½ tablespoons peanut butter and ½ serving of crackers
- 1½ tablespoons peanut butter on a sliced apple or small banana
- 2 wedges Laughing Cow light spreadable cheese on ½ serving of crackers, carrots, and celery sticks
- 1 ounce reduced-fat hard cheese (like Cabot 50 percent reduced fat) with ½ serving of crackers
- 1 small whole wheat pita filled with 2 tablespoons hummus
- Half of a ham-and-cheese sandwich with mustard on whole wheat bread or a small whole wheat pita
- Half of an English muffin topped with grated part-skim mozzarella, heated in the toaster oven
- 1 slice of whole grain bread with 1 slice of reduced-fat cheese, heated in the toaster oven
- 6 ounces light yogurt and ½ serving of nuts
- 1 light or plain yogurt mixed with 2 tablespoons low-fat granola
- ½ serving of nuts and one fruit
- 1–2 slices of turkey rolled into a small tortilla or stuffed into a small pita with lettuce, tomato, avocado, or sliced red peppers
- 1 hard-boiled egg and 1 slice whole wheat toast
- 6 ounces nonfat or low-fat Greek yogurt
- ½ cup high-fiber cereal with 4 ounces skim or 1 percent milk
- 1 reduced-fat cheddar stick or string cheese with ½ serving of crackers or a fruit

- ¾ cup homemade trail mix made with 2 cups high-fiber cereal, ⅓ cup chopped nuts, and ⅓ cup dried fruit (makes about 3½ servings)
- 1 hard granola bar coated with 2 teaspoons peanut butter

A warning: Be careful with cereal bars and chewy granola bars as they're often low in protein and high in sugar (check the nutrition facts on the packaging—you'd be surprised how much added sugar is in these "healthy" snack foods). Also, keep in mind that calorie-controlled, pre-portioned snack packs only save you calories if you eat just one. These packs may be a better option for an occasional after-meal treat (be sure to factor the carbs into your carb-distributed plan).

Dinner's Ready!

As you prepare for your final meal of the day, embrace these prediabetes diet plan rules:

1. The number-one rule: don't eat it too late! This tends to encourage reactive overeating at night, which can also kill your appetite for breakfast. A 2013 study from the *International Journal of Obesity* suggests that people who avoid excessive late-day eating may be more successful with weight loss.[2]

2. Establish the habit of preparing balanced-plate dinners most nights as one of your most important behavioral tasks. Even if you're not yet convinced you need to do this for yourself, if you have children, model healthy eating for them. Children learn what they live. Unhealthy behaviors—like eating out all the time and not eating until you're starving—is a recipe for overeating and becoming overweight.

3. Cook in bulk so your efforts extend beyond one meal. If you're going to make chicken or pork chops, make enough for three meals. Some people are afraid to do this because they worry they'll just eat more. Try storing the extra portions before dinner to make this less likely. Make enough brown rice at the beginning of the week so you'll have extra to reheat in the microwave. Stock your refrigerator with frozen vegetables so you'll always have something if you run out of fresh veggies. Make chili, soups, stews, and other meals you can prepare in a big batch and freeze in single-serving portions. All you have to do is thaw, reheat, and serve with a salad.

4. Preserve your favorite go-to recipes. If cookbooks intimidate you, buy a photo album and preserve behind plastic your favorite recipes from magazines, friends, and online recipe sites. This gives you something to flip through the next time you need reminding of what you might like for dinner!

5. Don't let vegetables be an afterthought. Although it's natural to plan your meal around the protein part, remember that half your plate should be vegetables. Having them in your house in fresh, frozen, or canned form is key to making them a priority.

6. Consider a trial of home-delivered groceries. Shopping often enough can be a challenge, and home delivery of fresh fruits and vegetables and other staples is a great option for busy people.

7. Take a cooking class to gain confidence in your culinary skills. Investigate options at a local adult education center or culinary school.

What are the usual mistakes people make about dinner?

- Eating too late or eating too little over the day. Both are classic set-ups for overeating at night.

- Not carving out time to shop during the week, so there's nothing to make for dinner.

- Couples too easily defaulting to "let's just eat out." It's tough to be the one leading the charge to eat more meals at home, but readiness to change doesn't always occur simultaneously for people in a relationship. Be optimistic that if you lead, your partner will eventually follow—or at least be supportive.

The Dinner Menu

Once you have an understanding of the carb-counting concept, there's a lot of flexibility with what you can eat for dinner. It's all about portions. Let's go back to the balanced-plate idea.

Populate a quarter of your plate with protein. If you eat off a ten-inch plate (or smaller), a quarter of the plate should equal a roughly 3- to 4-ounce cooked portion of meat, poultry, or seafood. If your calorie needs are higher (if you're male or extremely physically active, for instance), you may be able to eat up to 6 ounces of protein. To control calories, limit foods that are fried or in a cream or butter sauce to occasional use only. It's fine to pan-fry in a small amount of oil (2 tablespoons oil used in a recipe that serves four is only 1½ teaspoons of oil per person), or look for "light" versions of traditionally fatty recipes in cooking magazines or recipe websites. You may figure out how to make a lower-fat version of your favorite dish! In general, opt for grilled, baked, steamed, poached, or stewed meat, poultry, or seafood recipes. Lean sources of protein include any kind of seafood, white meat poultry without the skin, and lean cuts of meat with the words "loin," "round," "flank," "select," "choice," or "90 percent lean" or leaner in the name.

Consider using a slow-cooker. Preparing dinner can be as simple as layering chicken over a bed of cut vegetables, adding some chicken broth, and seasoning with your favorite herbs and spices. There are loads of slow-cooker recipes on the Internet. Be wary of high-fat ingredients.

Spice up your life. One challenge for the novice cook is figuring out how to add flavor to recipes without adding too much fat. Fortunately, as American cuisine has gotten more multicultural, we've become exposed to a greater variety of seasonings. Beyond such traditional herbs and spices as basil, oregano, dill, thyme, rosemary, and tarragon, there are countless delicious herb and spice blends, like Italian and poultry seasonings, Asian spice mixes, and spicy Southwestern and Indian blends for those who like to add a little kick to their food. If you need some inspiration, one great resource is Penzey's Spices (www.penzeys.com), a mostly mail-order business that sells high-quality spices and provides hundreds of recipes on their website (and in their free catalog). Start simple by rubbing a new spice onto your chicken breast before baking. You may be a more creative cook before you know it!

Experiment with starch choices. Covering a quarter (to a third, if needed) of your plate with a starch choice will help you avoid that deprived feeling, but it will also be a reasonable enough portion to avoid spiking your demand for insulin. Higher-fiber grains are brown rice, quinoa, whole wheat pasta, and whole grain bread. If you don't like brown rice, try cooking it in broth to add flavor or opt for basmati white rice, which has a lower glycemic index than long grains. Colorful starchy vegetables—like sweet potatoes, yams, winter squash, corn, peas, and dried beans—are super-healthy stand-ins, providing both the carbs we crave and an assortment of healthy nutrients. You can take nonstarchy vegetables and make a gratin using reduced-fat cheese, where the bread crumb top crust is the starch but the bulk of the recipe is low carb. There's also the amazingly tasty mashed cauliflower that many substituted for mashed potatoes in the low-carb diet days. Many versions of this mashed cauliflower recipe exist on the Internet, but be wary of those with too much added fat.

Go vegetarian and combine the protein and starch parts of your plate. Rice and beans. Tofu, rice, and stir-fried vegetables. Vegetarian chili and brown rice. A veggie burger on a whole grain bun. An egg, veggie sausage patty, and whole wheat English muffin sandwich. They're all plant protein and starch combos. You are adding some carbs in the form of plant protein, but beans, tofu, veggie burgers, and other meat substitutes also contain fiber, which helps mute their glycemic effect. There are many delicious and filling options in this category.

Salad for Supper

For many people, a salad consists of iceberg lettuce and salad dressing. What you want from a salad are phytonutrients—plant chemicals that circulate around the body promoting good health—of which pale iceberg lettuce has few. You want your salad to be colorful: dark leafy lettuce (romaine, green leaf, red leaf, Boston lettuce); spinach or baby spinach; green, red, orange, or yellow peppers; tomatoes; banana, jalapeño, or red roasted peppers; avocado; artichokes; carrots; cucumbers; beets; olives; broccoli; and cauliflower. The list goes on and on.

Protein can add flavor and texture to your salad, and is absolutely necessary if you want it to be a filling meal. Try the following:

- Grilled chicken
- Canned chicken or tuna
- Leftover meat, poultry, or seafood
- Beans (kidney, garbanzo, black, pinto)—rinsed, canned beans are fine
- Tofu cubes, soy nuts, edamame
- Reduced-fat shredded cheese
- Eggs and egg whites
- Small amounts of strong-tasting cheese, like feta, blue, and gorgonzola

A sprinkling of healthy fat in the salad adds flavor and helps you absorb the many fat-soluble phytonutrients in plant foods. These are some great alternatives:

- Nuts and seeds
- Avocado
- Olives and olive or canola oil
- Reduced-fat salad dressing, oil and vinegar, or a very small amount of full-fat dressing well tossed throughout the salad

Fresh or dried fruit can add flavor and texture in salads. These fruits make for some sweet additions:

- Dried cranberries or raisins
- Mandarin oranges
- Chunked pineapple
- Cut-up apples or pears

You can almost feel how filling a salad with all of these ingredients would be. Pair it with a whole grain roll or pita and a glass of 1 percent or skim milk and you have an incredibly nutritious, filling, balanced-plate dinner.

Balanced-Plate Dinner Ideas

Remember, nonstarchy vegetables count as zero carbs. With our goal of eating at least two fruits a day, note that some of the dinner options include fruit. Others include the occasional dessert, although try not to have dessert every night (to save calories). With all meal options, and certainly at dinnertime, limit fat used in cooking to 2 tablespoons in a pan and added fat at the table to 2 teaspoons (using Smart Balance, Olivio, or other trans fat–free tub spread). Try these dinners as is, or use them as a blueprint to mix and match your favorite foods, now that you have a sense of the carb-counting principles.

Balanced-Plate Dinner Ideas

DINNER CHOICE	CARBS (GRAMS)	
3–6 ounces cooked fish, poultry, or lean meat	0	**45 grams total** *(Note: It's okay to exempt the orange wedges from the carb count.)*
1 cup cooked sweet potato	30	
1 cup steamed asparagus	0	
Side spinach salad with almonds and mandarin oranges	0	
8 ounces skim or 1 percent milk	15	
2 teaspoons heart-healthy spread	0	
3–6 ounces grilled or stir-fried shrimp	0	**75 grams total**
1 cup brown or basmati rice	45	
1 cup steamed green beans with sesame seeds	0	
8 ounces skim or 1 percent milk	15	
12 cherries	15	
2 teaspoons heart-healthy spread	0	
3–4 ounces chicken cacciatore	0	**45 grams total** *(Note: Be sure to measure the whole wheat pasta—it's easy to go overboard!)*
Tomatoes, onions, peppers in the sauce	0	
1 cup whole wheat pasta	45	
Salad with greens, tomatoes, cucumbers, olives, and carrots	0	
1–2 tablespoons low-fat dressing	0	
Water or sugar-free beverage	0	
3–4 ounces sirloin steak or pork loin chop	0	**45 grams total** *(Note: Be sure to measure the yogurt!)*
Half large baked potato	30	
½ cup steamed broccoli	0	
½ cup steamed carrots	0	
2 teaspoons heart-healthy spread	0	
Water or sugar-free beverage	0	
½ cup low-fat frozen yogurt	15	
1 cup kidney or black beans	30	**60 grams total**
⅔ cup brown or basmati rice	30	
1 cup sautéed brussels sprouts	0	
Water or sugar-free beverage	0	
Sugar-free gelatin or frozen dessert	0	

Balanced-Plate Dinner Ideas, continued

DINNER CHOICE	CARBS (GRAMS)	
2 cups salad greens	0	
Tomatoes, peppers, beets, olives, onions, carrots, artichokes, and quarter avocado	0	
3 ounces grilled or canned chicken	0	
½ cup garbanzo beans (chickpeas)	15	
2 tablespoons dried cranberries	15	**60 grams total**
1 tablespoon sunflower seeds	0	
1 tablespoon low-fat salad dressing	0	
Half naan bread or one (six-inch) whole wheat pita	30	
2 teaspoons heart-healthy spread	0	
Water or sugar-free beverage	0	
Two slices whole grain bread	30	
Two slices turkey, ham, or lean roast beef	0	
1 teaspoon light mayonnaise	0	
1 teaspoon honey mustard*	0	
1 cup tomato soup	15	**60 grams total** *(*Free food because of the small portion.)*
Salad with greens, grape tomatoes, cucumbers, peppers, and onions (or other vegetables on hand)	0	
2 tablespoons low-fat salad dressing	0	
5 chocolate "kisses"	15	
Water or sugar-free beverage	0	
2 cups of beef stew (made with lean beef, carrots, potatoes, and other vegetables)	30	
1 cup steamed broccoli	0	**45 grams total**
8 ounces skim or 1 percent milk	15	
Half (12-inch) pizza, cheese or veggie	60	
Large salad with at least five veggies and ½ cup kidney or garbanzo beans	15	
2 tablespoons low-fat salad dressing	0	**75 grams total**
Sugar-free ice pop	0	
Water or sugar-free beverage	0	
Three or four 1-ounce meatballs made with 90 percent lean ground beef	0	
1 cup whole wheat pasta	45	**60 grams total** *(Measure the pasta. Use no-added-sugar or low-sugar tomato sauce.)*
Tomato sauce	0	
1 cup steamed broccoli and cauliflower	0	
8 ounces skim or 1 percent milk	15	

Balanced-Plate Dinner Ideas, continued

DINNER CHOICE	CARBS (GRAMS)	
1½ cups chili with ground turkey and beans	30	
⅓ cup brown rice	15	
2 tablespoons grated Parmesan cheese	0	**60 grams total**
1 cup steamed green beans	0	
8 ounces skim or 1 percent milk	15	
Sugar-free ice pop	0	
Two (6-inch) whole wheat tortillas	30	
3–6 ounces 90 percent lean ground beef or turkey breast, seasoned	0	
½ cup kidney or other beans	15	
½ cup part-skim grated Mexican cheese mix	0	**60 grams total**
Shredded lettuce, diced tomatoes, slices of avocado	0	*(*Free in this amount.)*
¼ cup salsa*	0	
1 tablespoon taco sauce*	0	
1 cup cantaloupe cubes	15	
Water or sugar-free beverage	0	

Eating More Plant Foods

Whether your goal is to reverse prediabetes, lose weight, or lower your risk for heart disease and cancer (or all of the above), an important part of every health-promoting diet is to eat a more plant-based diet. Here are some helpful tips to work more fruits and vegetables into your meals and snacks.

Keep an open mind. Fruits and vegetables you may not have liked earlier in life may be more appealing now. Go ahead, try something new!

Make time to shop. Having fresh produce in your home—and stored where you can see it—serves as a reminder to eat more. Studies show people eat more fruit if it's left out in sight, so keep fruit in a bowl on the kitchen table or counter. Store vegetables on the eye-level refrigerator shelves where they're visible, as opposed to shoved down below in the crisper where you may forget about them.

Do some quick prep. When you get home from the market, immediately cut up fruits into fruit salad or chop fresh vegetables and store them in a resealable bag so all you have to do is pull them out, wash, and cook.

Consider veggies throughout the day. Think of them as something to eat at lunch and snack time as well as at dinner.

Squeeze some in by lunchtime. Try to fit in at least two servings of fruits and vegetables by lunch. This timing increases the odds that you'll get in the recommended minimum of five to seven servings of fruits and vegetables by the end of the day. In general, a serving is ½ cup cooked or 1 cup raw, or a piece of fruit about the size of a tennis ball.

Here are some meal-specific ideas for adding more plants to your plate.

Breakfast. Add fresh fruit to your breakfast. Try a sliced banana or berries in your cereal or oatmeal, or some melon or an orange alongside your toast or eggs. Blend up a fruit smoothie with frozen fruit and plain yogurt. Add sautéed vegetables—like onions, peppers, or broccoli—to scrambled eggs or an omelet.

Snacks. Have some fruit as a midmorning snack. Leave an apple, banana, or pear on your desk at work so you remember you have it. Snack on yogurt with berries or dried fruit mixed in, sliced fruit dipped in peanut butter, or baby carrots dipped in hummus.

Lunch and dinner. Throw extra frozen vegetables into soups, stews, and casseroles. Add rinsed canned beans to salads and canned soups for added protein and fiber. When dining out, choose bean soups and veggie wraps, light on the dressing. Remember that salad bars offer good opportunities to sample new vegetables. Throw last night's cold leftover vegetables into a salad for lunch. Add frozen vegetables (broccoli, cauliflower, carrots) to tomato sauces to help fill you up without needing an extra serving of pasta. Stuff a baked potato with canned diced tomatoes, peppers, onions, steamed broccoli, and reduced-fat grated cheese. Load wrap sandwiches with greens, red peppers, and grated carrots.

Part 3

REVERSING PREDIABETES THROUGH WEIGHT LOSS, A HEART-HEALTHY DIET, AND EXERCISE

8

The Prediabetes-Obesity Connection

Obesity is a major risk factor for prediabetes and type 2 diabetes. While in the past we largely thought of excess body fat as simply stored calories, we now know that fat cells release fatty acids, hormones, inflammatory chemicals, and other substances that can aggravate insulin resistance. As such, weight loss should be a first-line focus for anyone with prediabetes who is overweight or obese. The good news is that studies indicate even modest weight loss has been shown to improve insulin resistance. Trimming calories and excess dietary fat, getting some regular physical activity, and ongoing follow-up with a registered dietitian or other supportive health care professional is the ideal combination for achieving the 7 percent weight loss research suggests may help prevent or control type 2 diabetes.[1] A single ideal dietary plan for weight loss for someone with prediabetes has not been determined, most likely because no one approach is going to work for all people. We all have different genetics, backgrounds, preferences, and priorities. But studies have found that both low-carb and low-fat calorie-controlled diets, as well as Mediterranean-type diets, can be effective at promoting weight loss in the short term. Maintaining weight loss long term is what really matters for managing and perhaps even reversing prediabetes, and regardless of dietary approach, increased physical activity and behavior modification are critical for helping to keep those lost pounds off.[2]

Research recently published in the *Journal of the American Medical Association* suggests that a diet with a low glycemic load (about 40 percent of calories from carbohydrate, 35 percent from fat, and 25 percent from protein) may provide an advantage for maintaining weight loss, particularly for people who are known to be insulin resistant. A 2012 study from Boston's Children's Hospital found that a diet moderate in carbohydrates that emphasized foods with a low glycemic load may promote more weight and body-fat loss than a low-fat diet in those with insulin resistance (as determined by high levels of insulin in the blood thirty minutes after an oral glucose tolerance test).[3] This study is far from conclusive but does offer insight into the probable need to pay attention to carbs when trying to lose weight with insulin resistance.

Getting Real: Evaluating Your Weight

Although more weight loss is better, losing just 7 percent of your current body weight may be enough to prevent or control type 2 diabetes. For a 250-pound person, this means losing as little as 18 pounds may be enough to reverse prediabetes. Just 7 percent. That's pretty astounding. I'm reinforcing this point for two reasons:

1. Many people skim over statistics because it's not their thing, and as a result they don't truly understand what they mean.

2. Even if your body mass index (BMI; more on this shortly) is still quite a bit above the "desirable" range, I want to make it exceedingly clear: *you can lose a very reasonable amount of weight and get significant health results.*

Let's look at another example. A 230-pound woman who is five feet six inches tall has a BMI of 37. If she loses just 16 pounds, she'll have lost 7 percent of her starting body weight, bringing her to 214. According to the BMI charts, she now has a BMI of 34.5. This still puts her in the obese category (those with BMIs of 30 or greater), but that's down from her initial BMI of 37 when she weighed 230. She is still overweight, but she'll reap meaningful health benefits from losing this modest amount of weight. It's very important to appreciate this benefit. The pressure of feeling the need to reduce your weight to where your BMI is "normal," or below 25 (which in our example would require the 230-pound woman to get down to 150 pounds), can be enough to discourage many people from even trying.

The tough sell here is that in our society we're conditioned to feel like we're supposed to go from overweight to slim when we "diet." Many people rate their success based on how they look versus how much healthier they are after weight loss. It's not that we don't appreciate the health benefits of weight loss; it's just generally not the main attraction. Given the challenges involved in losing weight, we need to expand our definition of success so we can appreciate the benefits of losing an amount of weight that's reasonable for many people to achieve. This is particularly important for preventing diabetes. By all means, think big. But don't lose sight of the value of small successes.

BMI Explained

When figuring out your health goals, start by evaluating your weight. The body mass index was created as a new way of assessing a healthy weight (see the chart opposite from the National Institutes of Health). The BMI is calculated using a person's height and weight and is considered a reliable indicator of body fatness. BMI does not measure body fat directly, but research has shown that BMI correlates to direct measures of body fat, such as underwater weighing, which is considered the gold standard for measuring body composition. BMI is used to determine at what weight you may begin to experience an increase in health problems. The number is calculated using a complex calculation (weight in kilograms divided by height in meters squared), but anyone with Internet access can bypass the math by using an online BMI calculator. These are two sources:

- Centers for Disease Control and Prevention, www.cdc.gov/ healthyweight/assessing/bmi/
- Department of Health and Human Services and the National Institutes of Health, www.nhlbisupport.com/bmi/

Body Mass Index and Weight Status

BMI	WEIGHT STATUS
Less than 18.5	Underweight
18.5–24.9	Normal
25–29.9	Overweight
30 and above	Obese

	Normal						Overweight					Obese										Extreme Obesity			
BMI	19	20	21	22	23	24	25	26	27	28	29	30	31	32	33	34	35	36	37	38	39	40	41	42	43
Height (inches)	Body Weight (pounds)																								
58	91	96	100	105	110	115	119	124	129	134	138	143	148	153	158	162	167	172	177	181	186	191	196	201	205
59	94	99	104	109	114	119	124	128	133	138	143	148	153	158	163	168	173	178	183	188	193	198	203	208	212
60	97	102	107	112	118	123	128	133	138	143	148	153	158	163	168	174	179	184	189	194	199	204	209	215	220
61	100	106	111	116	122	127	132	137	143	148	153	158	164	169	174	180	185	190	195	201	206	211	217	222	227
62	104	109	115	120	126	131	136	142	147	153	158	164	169	175	180	186	191	196	202	207	213	218	224	229	235
63	107	113	118	124	130	135	141	146	152	158	163	169	175	180	186	191	197	203	208	214	220	225	231	237	242
64	110	116	122	128	134	140	145	151	157	163	169	174	180	186	192	197	204	209	215	221	227	232	238	244	250
65	114	120	126	132	138	144	150	156	162	168	174	180	186	192	198	204	210	216	222	228	234	240	246	252	258
66	118	124	130	136	142	148	155	161	167	173	179	186	192	198	204	210	216	223	229	235	241	247	253	260	266
67	121	127	134	140	146	153	159	166	172	178	185	191	198	204	211	217	223	230	236	242	249	255	261	268	274
68	125	131	138	144	151	158	164	171	177	184	190	197	203	210	216	223	230	236	243	249	256	262	269	276	282
69	128	135	142	149	155	162	169	176	182	189	196	203	209	216	223	230	236	243	250	257	263	270	277	284	291
70	132	139	146	153	160	167	173	181	188	195	202	209	216	222	229	236	243	250	257	264	271	278	285	292	299
71	136	143	150	157	165	172	179	186	193	200	208	215	222	229	236	243	250	257	265	272	279	286	293	301	308
72	140	147	154	162	169	177	184	191	199	206	213	221	228	235	242	250	258	265	272	279	287	294	302	309	316
73	144	151	159	166	174	182	189	197	204	212	219	227	235	242	250	257	265	272	280	288	295	302	310	318	325

Interpreting Your BMI

BMI interpretations are designed for people over age twenty. Because BMI is calculated using weight that includes both lean and fat mass, a small percentage of people may appear overweight because they have excess muscle, as might be the case with a competitive athlete. That would account for some people drifting into the overweight range. Most people with a BMI above 30, however, have excess body fat. Another limitation of BMI is that it's only one indicator of overall health—others being diet, activity level, and family and personal health history. Once you know your BMI, you can determine whether you're already at a healthy weight or are considered underweight, overweight, or obese.

The BMI ranges are based on the relationship between body weight and disease and death. Overweight and obese individuals are at increased risk for many health problems, including the following:

- Hypertension
- High LDL cholesterol, low HDL cholesterol, high levels of triglycerides in the blood

- Type 2 diabetes
- Heart disease
- Stroke
- Gallbladder problems
- Arthritis
- Sleep apnea and respiratory problems
- Some cancers (endometrial, breast, colon, possibly others)

Feeling overwhelmed and even a little defeated? Please don't. Let me repeat: *just because you can't imagine getting your BMI down to the below-25 range doesn't mean weight loss isn't worth it.* Losing just enough to reverse prediabetes is extremely valuable. Ask anyone with diabetes whether they'd rather invest their time working on diet and lifestyle change to avoid getting diabetes versus learning how to balance diet, activity, and medications to control their diabetes once they have it. The majority of people would wish they hadn't waited to make changes. Work on it now or work on it later—in both situations diet and activity habits have to change.

Failed Weight-Loss Approaches

Before we look at diet and lifestyle habits tied to lasting weight loss, let's review why historically many of our weight-loss approaches haven't worked. There have been countless "diets" to choose from over the years, most involving a sudden, dramatic change in what you eat. Some diets have recommended avoiding entire food groups (fats, carbs, white flour, gluten), whereas others have offered packaged foods so you don't have to think much about meal planning. Many plans have called for severe calorie restriction, maybe as low as 1,000 calories. Others go even lower, usually as part of a medically supervised diet that relies on protein-packed milk shakes. Regardless of the approach, what most of these fad diets have in common is radical dietary change, with the unspoken promise that if you just stick to the rules you will lose weight.

For many of us this translates into, "If I just behave and stop acting so weak around food, I'll be able to lose weight." The problem with that thinking is that most diets are doomed to fail because they threaten your body's internal instincts geared toward self-preservation. They don't focus enough on exercise and providing skills to make permanent change. Any dietary changes that cut your calories back will result in weight loss. We may know that what we're doing to lose weight can't possibly be maintained for the long haul, or shouldn't be because it's not healthy, but somehow we hold out hope that this new diet will be the one that doesn't result in our regaining the lost weight (often more than we lost in the first place). But think about it: If at the end of an overrestrictive diet you drift back to the diet and lifestyle habits that got you into trouble in the first place, why wouldn't you get the same result?

For these and many other reasons, we've got to stop thinking about "dieting" and start framing weight loss as something that happens when we adopt healthier habits, permanently. I know, very unsexy, but it's true. The things that you can do to reverse your prediabetes, and in general help you feel physically and mentally better every day, are the same things that should result in weight loss if practiced consistently. And it is never a bad thing to think about managing your blood sugar versus losing pounds. I've had many clients who, after achieving a better understanding of what it takes to control insulin resistance, have lost weight for the first time in a long time, all while avoiding the psychological baggage that goes along with "dieting."

Mind-Set Intervention: Weight Loss Is Possible!

Weight-loss dieting tends to bring out the worst in us, psychologically speaking. When contemplating yet another weight-loss attempt, many of us spiral through thoughts like these: *I've tried this so many times before and failed, so why bother again? My body is just incapable of weight loss. I'm hopelessly addicted to food. I have no self-control. I'm so uncoordinated, and exercise is so uncomfortable.* Focusing on painful past experiences is natural, but as much as possible, try to think of it in this way: you can either stick with your current habits and risk becoming diabetic, or start today deconstructing your old, unhealthy habits and replace them with healthier ones. The beauty of the prediabetes diet plan is that it can help you lose weight by giving you a new focus. It's not really about weight loss—it's about your health. Instead of "don't eat this, don't do that," you're changing behaviors to help improve your insulin resistance. You still end up trimming calories by eating smaller amounts more frequently, watching your portions, and being more active on a daily basis, but the focus is on the immediate response of controlling blood glucose and insulin levels. This is very different from the typical "dieting" approach of psyching yourself up for a process that will painfully rob you of many of the foods you love.

Science and Successful Losers

In 1994, Dr. Rena Wing of Brown University and Dr. James Hill of the University of Colorado founded the National Weight Control Registry (NWCR), which has been tracking the behaviors of more than ten thousand people who have lost significant amounts of weight and successfully kept it off. Registry participants have maintained a weight loss of at least thirty pounds for at least one year.[4] Many weight-loss programs are able to consistently produce weight losses of 7 to 10 percent of initial body weight at the end of six to twelve months, but many of those people regain the weight within a relatively short period of time. Why is it so difficult to lose weight and keep it off? Although we don't have all the answers to this question, some factors we know play a role include physiological, psychological, and behavioral changes that can be tough to sustain. Physiological changes that occur during weight loss, such as a decline in the body's metabolic rate and changes in thyroid and hunger hormone activity, can make it tougher to feel satisfied and therefore easier to eat too much. Psychological and behavioral changes—boredom with food choices, decreased motivation over time after the thrill of losing the weight is gone—can also be tough to sustain.

What is clear is that losing weight and keeping it off requires permanent, sustainable changes as well as ongoing support from friends, family, health care providers, and group programs. Let's look at some data from the National Weight Control Registry. The NWCR recruits participants who are at least eighteen years old. Eighty percent of registry members are women, 20 percent are men. Members provide information yearly via questionnaires on eating habits, activity patterns, and weight-control strategies. Demographically, NWCR participants have a lot in common. They are 95 percent Caucasian, 82 percent college educated, and 64 percent married. Efforts are under way to diversify the gender, ethnic, and socioeconomic status of the group. The average woman is forty-five years old and currently weighs 145 pounds, while the average man is forty-nine years old and currently weighs 190 pounds.

Here's the inspiring part: Before starting to lose weight, the average BMI of NWCR participants was well into the obese range (a BMI greater than 30). Upon entry into the registry, the average member had lost sixty-six pounds (the range is thirty to three hundred pounds lost!) and kept it off for an average of 5.5 years. About 45 percent of participants lost weight on their own; 55 percent participated in group programs or individual counseling with a therapist or dietitian.

Helpful Weight-Loss Strategies

The vast majority of NWCR participants (89 percent) used both diet and physical activity to lose weight. Just 10 percent changed only their diet, and 1 percent changed only their level of activity. As for dietary changes, the three most common weight-loss techniques were the following:

- Limiting intake of foods associated with weight gain, like sweets and fatty foods, including desserts
- Decreasing portion sizes of all foods
- Counting calories (about 50 percent count calories or fat grams)

For physical activity, 92 percent of NWCR participants exercised at home, with walking and aerobic dancing more common in women and competitive sports and weightlifting more common in men. A large chunk, about 40 percent, had an exercise "buddy," and about 31 percent exercised as part of a group. Equally impressive are the participants' reported quality-of-life scores:

- Almost all participants (95.3 percent) reported improvements in their quality of life (both physical and psychological)
- Almost all (92.4 percent) experienced improved energy and mobility, making physical activity more possible
- Mood improved as well, with 91.4 percent of participants reporting decreases in symptoms of depression

This last point is particularly important. Studies show that weight regain is significantly more common in people who feel more depressed (and therefore prone to uncontrolled eating, often in response to stress).

Maintenance Strategies

When it comes to weight-loss maintenance, there were many common strategies among the losers. In terms of what they ate, though not perfect, successful losers seem a bit better than the average American at eating according to health experts' recommendations.[5] As with many statistics, these are averages, so, for example, there would definitely be a range of intakes of carbohydrates, protein, and fat in their diets. Here are some strategies of successful losers.

They're constantly vigilant about what they eat. Calorie intake is maintained at a fairly low level—on average about 1,400 calories. The NWCR founders speculate these low numbers may reflect the fact that many of the participants reported they were still trying to lose weight. Also, studies show that people, particularly those who are overweight, are notorious for underreporting food intake, so a reported intake of 1,400 calories may actually be higher.

They watch their fat intake. Average fat intake for the successful losers is reported at about 24 percent of total calories (definitely a low-fat diet), or about 45 grams of fat a day. More recent participants reported a fat intake of about 29 percent, likely reflecting the recent popularity of low-carb diets.

They're mindful of carb and protein intake as well. Carb intake has declined over the past few years for NWCR participants but still averages about 53 percent of daily calories, or 182 grams of carb a day. Protein intake is about 19 percent of calories on average for these folks, or about 64 grams per day.

They make it a point to eat their veggies. Registry participants eat an average of four servings a day, and they eat more fiber from fruits, vegetables, and beans than from grains.

They don't forget to eat breakfast. Breakfast is a must among 78 percent of NWCR participants, which supports reams of research tying breakfast intake with weight loss (and less eating at night).

They eat more meals at home than out. Most participants reported preparing meals at home, eating outside the home only three times a week—and they rarely ate fast food.

Eating patterns matter. The average NWCR member eats about five times a day, suggesting they make efforts to stay ahead of their hunger to avoid overeating. They also work hard to maintain their calorie-control efforts on both weekdays and weekends as well as around the holidays (which can be times of overindulgence for many of us).

They monitor their weight on a regular basis. More than 75 percent of registry participants weigh themselves more than once a week. They say that monitoring their weight helps guide their diet and physical activity choices, which allows them to get right on any regain when it's only a pound or two.

Exercise plays a major role. About 76 percent of them reported walking, 20 percent lift weights, and 20 percent cycle, for an average of about sixty minutes a day. (These are moderate-intensity activities. According to government guidelines, sixty minutes of moderate activity a day can be replaced with thirty minutes of intense activity a day, like running or high-intensity aerobics.) Time spent on physical activity comes at the expense of "screen time." The average registry member watches only six to ten hours of TV, compared with twenty-eight hours per week for the average American.

What's clear from member feedback is that they spend a substantial amount of time and energy on these strategies, and they strive to be as consistent as possible. When NWCR members do begin to regain weight, it's most likely to happen in the early stages of maintenance and is most often associated with drifting from these proven strategies. On the positive side, participants report that it gets easier to maintain weight loss over time. Once they've maintained a weight loss for two to five years, their chances of long-term success increase greatly.

The Outlook of Successful Losers

Losing weight and keeping it off is challenging but not impossible. Weight loss positively affects every physical and emotional quality-of-life indicator. It requires support from others—be it family, friends, health care providers, or support groups—and research suggests that face-to-face support is best. Others may find what they need from an online source, like a weight-loss website, a smartphone app, or an online chat room (see the Resources section at the back of the book for some suggestions). Maintaining weight loss can be even more challenging, as it requires some swimming upstream against social norms. Eating out too often can make it hard to control your calorie intake. Too much time spent on the computer or watching TV can monopolize time that could otherwise be spent being physically active.

The ultimate ambition of the National Weight Control Registry is to teach aspiring "losers" skills that may help them succeed long term.

The NWCR founders' STOP Regain study recruited people who had lost at least 10 percent of their body weight over the previous two years and taught them the habits of the NWCR participants in weekly meetings for one month, followed by monthly meetings for eighteen months. The results were compelling: compared to a group who had no intervention, the STOP Regain program participants regained significantly less weight.[6]

Other research has looked at the emotional aspects at play in those who've achieved lasting weight loss. Registered dietitian Anne M. Fletcher, author of *Thin for Life: Ten Keys to Success from People Who Have Lost Weight and Kept It Off*, which captures the strategies of more than two hundred adults who have maintained weight loss, says: "These 'masters' of former weight problems recognize that there's no such thing as perfection when it comes to weight control. When they 'slip'—for instance, eat in a way they hadn't intended or miss a day of exercise—they don't berate themselves. Instead, they prevent such lapses from becoming full-blown relapses by keeping it in perspective and picking up right where they left off."

"Masters" of weight control seem to be resilient and able to learn from past experiences. Fletcher found it's not uncommon for those who ultimately succeed to have lost weight and regained it numerous times in the past. "Rather than let these attempts serve as cruel reminders of failure," Fletcher advises, "it's more useful to view past dieting efforts as learning opportunities, to identify what did and didn't work for you in the past." She suggests making two lists: one of strategies that worked for you in past dieting attempts (for example, getting up to eat breakfast or walking the dog after work), and another of strategies that did not work (such as eating grapefruit with every meal or getting up to go swimming at 5 a.m.). Then employ only those strategies that truly worked in the past. You've got to make sustainable change.

Comparing Recommendations: Prediabetes Diet Plan and NWCR

Although the prediabetes diet plan requires some fine-tuning to manage insulin resistance (the focus of part 4 of this book), if you compare the plan to the NWCR's recommendations, you'll notice from the chart (opposite) that there's quite a bit of overlap. As you can see, there isn't one diet and lifestyle strategy for managing prediabetes and another one for

Comparing Recommendations:
The Prediabetes Diet Plan and NWCR Strategies

PREDIABETES DIET PLAN	NWCR RECOMMENDATIONS AND STRATEGIES
Spread carbs out over three meals and one to three snacks per day.	Eat an average of four to five times per day.
Cover half your plate with vegetables.	Eat four or more servings of vegetables daily.
Start the day with a protein-containing breakfast.	Eat breakfast daily.
Eat proactively to stay ahead of hunger.	Be continuously vigilant about portions and control portion sizes.
Budget out time each week to shop and plan meals to control choices.	Prepare most of your own meals.
Budget out time for daily activity to help manage your insulin resistance.	Be moderately active for sixty minutes daily.
Eat carbohydrates in moderation; don't overrestrict.	Eat carbohydrates in moderation; don't overrestrict.
Limit your fat intake to help control calories.	Follow a low-fat diet.
Eat protein in moderation—enough to help you feel full but not so much that you're getting too many calories.	Eat protein in moderation.
Control your food environment to limit temptations.	Limit eating out to three times weekly.
Focus on the positive; learn and move on from lapses.	Lapses are opportunities to learn, not evidence of weakness or failure.

weight loss. They both accomplish the same thing! If weight loss isn't your goal—not all people with prediabetes are overweight—you may need to increase lean protein and healthy fat intake to help fill the void left by trimming carbohydrate calories. Or you may need to add an extra snack. In any case, the goal of the prediabetes diet plan is to kill multiple birds with one stone (manage insulin resistance, reduce the risk for diabetes and heart disease, lose weight if necessary) without compromising the overall quality of the diet.

Protein and the Prediabetes Diet Plan

Whereas the NWCR folks average about 19 percent of their daily calories from protein, on the prediabetes diet plan you may need to eat a little more. According to the Dietary Guidelines for Americans, protein intake can healthfully provide anywhere from 10 to 35 percent of calories. The prediabetes diet meal plans offered in the back of the book suggest protein amounts within this healthy range. Choose lean options so your protein foods don't come packaged with a lot of fat.

When it comes to weight loss, research is mixed on whether eating more or less of any one nutrient (carbohydrate, protein, or fat) is more effective than any other. For example, one study from the Brigham and Women's Hospital in Boston of more than eight hundred people trying to lose weight tested four different diets. Each provided a different amount of calories from carbohydrate, protein, and fat. The fat ranged from 20 to 40 percent of daily calories, protein from 15 to 25 percent of daily calories, and carbohydrate from 35 to 65 percent of daily calories. All groups were offered individual and group support for two years. The results? All groups lost about the same amount of weight and experienced improvements in their blood lipid and insulin levels. Not surprisingly, attending the group sessions was strongly associated with weight-loss success.[7]

The take-home message is that cutting calories is what counts most, and there are many ways to accomplish that. What's unique about managing prediabetes, however, is we often have a two-pronged goal: weight loss and managing insulin response. Losing weight helps improve insulin resistance, but managing the insulin response can also make weight loss easier because having excess amounts of circulating insulin can make people hungry. Eating less carbohydrate in one sitting (particularly when it's paired with protein and a little healthy fat) will mute the body's post-meal demand for insulin. The goal of the prediabetes diet plan is to include enough protein in your day to help make eating less carbohydrate easier. From a physiological standpoint, there are several reasons why eating a bit more protein may help with weight loss:

- Protein increases fullness to a greater extent than carbohydrate, so including protein may make it easier to eat fewer calories at a meal or snack.
- Higher-protein diets are associated with increased thermogenesis (meaning your body burns more calories processing it), which in turn promotes a sense of fullness.
- In some people, eating more protein may help them retain more muscle while they're losing weight.[8]

Research backs up a protein-heavy approach. One study of women from the University of Illinois at Urbana-Champaign compared a higher-carb diet (with 68 grams of protein a day) with a higher-protein diet (with 125 grams of protein a day). After ten weeks the women lost about the same amount of weight, but the women in the higher-protein group lost significantly more body fat. The women with the higher-carb intake had higher insulin responses to meals and more postmeal hypoglycemia (which causes hunger), whereas the women in the higher-protein group reported a greater sense of fullness after meals and significant reductions in unhealthy blood triglyceride levels.[9] Please note that this doesn't support the use of a very low-carb, very high-protein diet for weight loss. We're talking balance here—trimming out most processed carbs in favor of whole grains, beans, fruits, and vegetables, and replacing some of those calories with a bit more protein, emphasizing lower-fat sources.

Ten Strategies for Weight Loss and Lifestyle Change

Beyond the recommendations of members of the National Weight Control Registry, I've found these ten strategies to be helpful for those trying to lose weight and make important lifestyle changes. The powerful strategies here are based more on behavior than food. Check off a few that might be helpful for you and start implementing them today.

Strategy #1: Learn How Your Body Works

Losing weight is difficult indeed. It's not that the body won't give up fat; it just doesn't like sudden, drastic cuts in calorie intake that may suggest an impending food shortage. The trick is to weed out a few calories here and there—by trimming portions, reducing fat intake (perhaps as simple as eating out less), opting for calorie-free beverages, and so forth—while still eating regularly throughout the day. Start by eating a satisfying breakfast, followed by a filling lunch that includes protein and plant foods, a satisfying carbohydrate-protein snack when your hunger starts to kick in right about midafternoon, and a dinner early enough in the evening that you're not ravenous when you sit down. Think of rating your hunger on a scale of 1 to 10—1 being "not hungry" and 10 being "starved." To avoid overeating, eat your next meal when your hunger is a 5 or 6—about halfway to "starved." If you wait until it's an 8 or a 10, you'll most likely to overreact and overeat when you finally get around to it. Also, while you're eating, pay attention to when you're no longer hungry, then try to stop eating. For example, if you only need half a granola bar to hold your hunger until the next meal, save the other half for your next snack.

The lesson here is to start thinking of eating as a positive thing. Going out of your way to eat may actually help you lose weight by helping your body feel it's okay to burn calories and help you stay ahead of your hunger. Digesting and processing food uses up about 10 percent of all the calories the body burns, so pump up your metabolic rate with breakfast, then continue to throw wood on the fire of your metabolism throughout the day by eating every four or five hours or so.

Strategy #2: Adjust Your Attitude

You're not a failure—and you won't fail in managing your prediabetes and losing weight if you follow these strategies. According to NWCR founder Dr. Rena Wing, "successful losers" are encouraged to view lapses as opportunities to learn, not as evidence of weakness or failure. I can't emphasize enough the importance of this. People who lose weight and keep it off accept there will be bumps in the road and try to develop strategies to manage them. One behavior pattern noted in those who lose weight and regain it is when they find themselves in a situation that veers them off track from their plan (like overeating with friends, indulging during a vacation, having a baby, grieving after someone dies—any life event that makes it hard to keep strictly to a program), they berate themselves with negative self-talk about weaknesses and past failures, and ultimately give up.

A more realistic reaction to bumps in the road is to analyze the situation to see how it could have been handled differently. Could the lapse have been prevented or lessened in any way? Successful losers reflect on what happened and why, determine whether the lapse was avoidable, and whether there's a strategy that could help them deal with that situation should it arise again.

Strategy #3: Keep a Food Journal

Studies have proven that food journaling helps keep people accountable for what they're eating. Buy a small colorful notebook that will get your

Lapses Happen; Now Move On

I call this the old cowboy strategy: Pick yourself up, dust yourself off, and get back in the saddle. No one eats perfectly all the time, and it's not necessary. Life isn't always predictable. You'll be thrown off track at times, so you've got to develop coping strategies. Here are a few curve balls life can throw at you along with strategies to help deal with them:

- Did you overeat at a restaurant? Maybe you were overhungry when you got there. Next time have a midafternoon carb-protein snack and perhaps a fruit on the way to the restaurant. This might make it easier to order the healthier option. Also, be careful who you dine with (eating out with overeaters may make it feel okay to step out of your healthy habits).
- Grabbed take-out on the way home? Maybe it was because you skipped your weekly trip to the supermarket. Schedule time to shop on the weekends so your cupboards aren't empty during the week.
- Skipped your trip to the gym because you forgot your workout clothes? Try packing a backup gym bag with an old pair of sneakers, shorts, and a T-shirt that you'll leave in your trunk for just this type of situation.
- Snacking from the work vending machine? Remind yourself to pack a snack from home the night before (along with a healthy lunch).
- Skipped breakfast because you were running late? Did you then overindulge at lunch? Set your clock a few minutes earlier so you have more time for a solid breakfast. Eating this meal (or not) sets the tone for the day: you're either eating proactively to stay ahead of your hunger or reactively in response to being overhungry.
- You're heading home for dinner and you haven't eaten any fruits or vegetables all day? Make a quick detour to the market on the way home to pick up some fresh or frozen vegetables, or assemble a take-home salad from the market. Be sure to pack fruits and veggies with your lunch and snacks for the next day. And store them where you can see them (on the kitchen counter, in a fruit bowl, and so on).
- Did you mindlessly eat too many cookies in front of the TV after dinner? Be realistic with yourself and keep impulse snacks out of the house. It's just easier that way. Instead, try a sugar-free gelatin, a cup of herbal tea, or a piece of gum while you work on deconditioning yourself from eating in front of the TV.

The bottom line is that you can deal with just about anything. Don't blow a lapse out of proportion! We all have imperfect meals, or days, or even weeks. What matters is that you learn from the experience and move on. Human beings are flawed. Don't set the bar too high.

attention. Some people prefer to log their food online or use a smartphone app (see the Resources section in the back of the book). Throughout the day, you'll record the time, food or beverage consumed, the amount, and anything else that might be helpful. Recording may make you think twice before you dive into that extra portion. You may be surprised about what you learn through keeping a food journal. It can help you identify problem areas and zone in on solutions. Keeping a food journal is also a way to keep your diet and behavior change goals in front of you. Every time you pull out your notebook or smartphone app, it's a reminder of what you're trying to accomplish.

Strategy #4: Avoid Overeating at Night

It's long been known that night-shift workers and those with "night eating syndrome" (an eating disorder where people, sometimes in their sleep, rise and eat at night) are prone to being overweight. After talking to thousands of people about weight loss over the years, I'm convinced that food distribution over the day matters. For people who are overweight, a similar pattern frequently emerges where food intake escalates as the day goes on. They may or may not eat breakfast or lunch, then find themselves starving by late afternoon and respond to it by diving into the vending machine or business meeting leftovers. They then go home and eat a large dinner and often snack again later in the evening, perhaps in front of the TV as they "unwind" from the busy day. In essence, they're eating less during the active time of the day and more in the evening, when the body is preparing for sleep. A recent study from Spain supports the potential benefits of eating more calories earlier in the day.[10] (In Spain the largest meal of the day tends to be midday.) Despite consuming the same number of calories, those who ate their main meal before 3 p.m. lost more weight over a twenty-week period.

The good news is people who tend to eat more in the evening often immediately start to lose weight once they switch to three meals and a snack or two over the day. Simply distributing their food more throughout the day seems to stimulate the body to let go of some reserves and helps them curb their food intake by staying ahead of their hunger.

Strategy #5: Budget Time for Self-Care

We're genetically hard-wired to be opportunistic eaters, and in modern society we're overexposed to food. For many of us, our daily schedule already feels congested, and making time to eat healthier and exercise feels like one more demand. But it's important to intentionally resist the temptation to eat whenever we're exposed to food and intentionally insert time for physical activity. If we designed a pie chart of all the things that demand our attention, it would likely include family, friends, work,

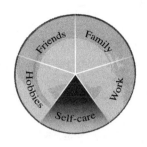

hobbies, pets, and other things that are important to us. To live a healthy life in today's culture, you need to carve out time to devote to self-care: buying healthy food, preparing and eating it; budgeting in time for physical activity; getting at least seven hours of sleep (the minimum amount researchers believe we need for good health); and managing stress (much of which might be taken care of by the addition of regular exercise!).

Making time for self-care isn't easy, but few things in life are more important than taking steps to protect your health. If you want a healthy lunch, pack it yourself and bring it to work. It's up to you to manage your food environment. Be proactive and populate your food world—your home, office, and car—with things you want to be eating. Keep out those things you know you should limit. If fruits, vegetables, whole grains, low-fat dairy, and lean proteins are closest at hand, that's what you're most likely to eat.

For those of you living with a partner, it's time for a little healthy selfishness! The other people in your house may not be ready to make change, but that doesn't mean you need to make your job harder by catering to different tastes. Healthy eating trumps junk food. Anything you do to improve the food environment at home almost always trickles down to others living there, which is especially important if you have children. Now may be a good time for a serious talk about who will do what to help nurture healthier eating habits in your home. If you and your partner are both busy and working, the odds of success for everyone will be much lower if all the responsibilities related to meal planning, shopping, and cooking fall on one person. If one of you is a better cook, maybe the other can find some healthier recipes and help out with shopping. Teamwork and support between couples and among family members is critical to success.

Strategy #6: Manage Your Hunger to Control Portions

Most of us overeat because we wait until we're overhungry before we eat. By that point all our caveman instincts are going to trigger us to eat fast, and way too much. It's easier to take more conscious decisions about what you eat—and how much—when your hunger level is a 5 or 6, not a 10. In essence, establish a pattern of proactive eating to prevent reactive overeating. To help us avoid overeating, we rely far too often on willpower and good intentions, both of which are genetically in short supply and neither of which is potent enough to help resist overeating when we're starving and exposed to too much food. Try adding a "hunger" column to your food journal where you record your hunger on this 1-to-10 scale. It may remind you to eat when you're at a 5 or 6.

Strategy #7: Make Losing Weight a Priority

Most of us can always find time to surf the Internet or watch TV. Maybe your new priority should be to postpone these activities until after you've taken a walk. Time to purchase and prepare food, exercise, sleep—even relaxation time—should be prioritized and budgeted into your day like all the other things you feel are important. This usually requires pushing back on all the people and things that make demands on your time (which can be especially difficult to do if you're the primary caregiver in the household). This is a critically important, proactive step—the time to do these things won't fall in your lap. Look at your schedule carefully and find the time to take care of yourself. Don't wait until your health problems have affected your quality of life before you get serious about this.

Strategy #8: Manage Your Expectations

No doubt, making healthy changes in your diet and losing weight is difficult, especially if you have years of dieting under your belt and have experienced weight-loss regain. Shaking off the negative thinking and overly ambitious expectations can be tough, but it's so important. To help you steer around some of the sticking points of the past, take these tips to heart:

- You can't change the past—you can only learn from it.
- Change is tough. Go easy on yourself. So what if it takes longer? Wading into the things you find challenging a little at a time may

feel less threatening (and is probably more sustainable for you) than jumping right into the deep end!

- Focus on getting through a single day. Setting a short-term goal and meeting it is a lot more empowering than focusing on a long-term goal that you don't even know is doable yet.
- Pay attention to what your body is telling you. Appreciate the numerous forms of positive feedback you get from eating better and exercising that have nothing to do with the number on the scale. Noticing all the little ways your body feels better is potent ammunition toward keeping you on track.
- If you bring high-risk foods into your house, in all likelihood you'll eat them. Very few people can eat just one potato chip!
- If you don't have a decent plan in place for when you get hungry, there is a very good chance you will not make the best choices. It's always better to eat proactively with foods you've prepared than reactively because you're overhungry.
- Focus on what you *can* eat, not just on what you think you can't!
- "Healthy eating" is more than simply avoiding junk food. If you add enough foods that are nutritious and filling into your day, there will be less room for the stuff that's not good for you.

Ultimately what helps any one individual lose weight is coming up with his or her own portfolio of things that work. Start by taking stock of your past experiences, including what has worked before (maybe shopping more consistently, exercising in the morning, not keeping ice cream in the house), and discard the things that didn't work (crash dieting, diet pills, excessive exercise). Review the strategies of the NWCR successful losers and start test-driving them to see what might work for you. Ascribe to the 80/20 rule: What you do 80 percent of the time represents your habits, the things you automatically default to when it comes to diet and exercise. Those are the habits you want to affirm. What happens the rest of the time represents days that aren't going "as usual." They don't carry anywhere near as much weight as your daily routines.

Strategy #9: Don't Go It Alone

Seek out support for your goals. A spouse, partner, family member, friend, or exercise buddy can be an invaluable asset. If you're a group person, join Weight Watchers (for local meetings or online membership) or TOPS (Take Off Pounds Sensibly, www.tops.org). As a nutritionist, I'm not a big fan of programs that require you to buy meal replacements, although that might be an option at the outset for some—as long as you understand the challenges of transitioning out of meal replacement drinks or bars to real food. Many people benefit from the personal coaching provided by registered dietitians (find one in your area on the Academy of Nutrition and Dietetics' website, www.eatright.org). By all means, if you need a therapist to help you shake free of emotional challenges that may hold you up, do it.

Because weight loss is so challenging, readiness is key. Even now, you may not be ready to jump into a weight-loss plan, but reading this book may move you a little farther along toward making positive, healthy changes. Renowned University of Rhode Island psychologist James Prochaska, author of *Changing for Good*, outlines five stages that people who are able to drop bad habits tend to progress through. These are known as the "transtheoretical model stages of change":[11]

- Precontemplation—change isn't on your radar
- Contemplation—you're thinking about it and researching options
- Preparation—setting the stage for change
- Action—you're doing it!
- Maintenance—you're working to make change stick

If you're not feeling ready to take charge of your health, manage your prediabetes, and lose weight, try to figure out what you need to do to establish that readiness. You can't just rely on willpower and good intentions to help you reverse your prediabetes. As I often tell my clients, in order for the very small amount of willpower and good intentions we naturally possess to be at all helpful when it comes to dealing with food, you need to develop a plan. A plan will help to avoid constantly dwelling in a chaotic food environment.

Strategy #10: Be Patient

The final strategy is perhaps the most important for long-term sustainability. Fad dieting is all about quick results, but it takes time for your body to get used to eating less food and for you to start experiencing the positive effects of increased physical activity. It takes determination and repetition to make shopping and planning meals a priority. These habits will eventually become second nature. Having faith that all your up-front work will eventually pay off is critical to staying focused and achieving long-term success.

9

Reducing Your Risk of Cardiovascular Disease

Because diabetes and cardiovascular disease are so closely linked, reducing your risk of diabetes can also lower your risk of having a heart attack or stroke. Consider these facts about heart disease, stroke, and high blood pressure from the American Diabetes Association: In 2004 "heart disease" was noted on 68 percent of diabetes-related death certificates among people age sixty-five or older. In 2004 "stroke" was noted on 16 percent of diabetes-related death certificates among people age sixty-five or older. Adults with diabetes have heart disease death rates about two to four times higher than adults without diabetes. The risk for stroke is two to four times higher among people with diabetes. During the period 2005 to 2008, of adults twenty years or older with self-reported diabetes, 67 percent had blood pressure greater than or equal to 140/90 mmHg or used prescription medications for hypertension.[1] These are staggering statistics.

The prediabetes diet plan is designed to help you manage insulin resistance, but the multipronged approach of controlling portions of carbs, watching fat intake (and eating healthier fats), choosing lean sources of protein, increasing activity, and eating more fruits, vegetables, and whole grains is one of the most potent things you can do to also control your blood cholesterol levels, manage your blood pressure, and lose weight. Along with diabetes, these conditions gobble up billions of health care dollars annually, imposing an unsustainable burden on the US health care system and negatively affecting quality of life for millions of Americans.

The Menace of Metabolic Syndrome

It is estimated that more than fifty million American men and women (approaching a fifth of the entire population) have metabolic syndrome, another condition driven by insulin resistance that is characterized by a collection of cardiovascular risk factors. According to the American Heart Association, metabolic syndrome occurs when a person has *three or more* of these cardiovascular risk factors:

- Abdominal obesity (excessive belly fat)
- Abnormal blood fat and cholesterol levels (high triglycerides, low HDL cholesterol, and high LDL cholesterol), which encourage plaque buildup in artery walls
- High blood pressure
- Insulin resistance
- Prothrombotic state, or a tendency for the blood to clot more easily
- Proinflammatory state, often diagnosed with a C-reactive protein test, a marker for inflammation in the blood

Although the primary goal of the prediabetes diet plan is to reduce insulin resistance and circulating levels of insulin, many of the risk factors for metabolic syndrome and heart disease could be positively affected by following the plan. Controlling insulin resistance with diet and exercise helps reduce belly fat. Avoiding saturated and trans fats and limiting intake of sweets helps improve triglyceride and cholesterol levels and enhance insulin sensitivity. Losing weight, exercising, and adding fruits, vegetables, whole grains, and small amounts of nuts to the diet can help lower blood pressure and reduce inflammation.[2] Increasing your intake of heart-healthy omega-3 fats can help thin the blood and reduce inflammation.

Numbers for a Healthy Heart

If you've found yourself checking off any of these criteria, it's important to know what your goal numbers for a healthy heart should be. While metabolic syndrome may require three or more criteria to make the diagnosis, if you suffer from even *one* of these criteria, controlling these numbers is an important part of protecting your cardiovascular system. Let's take a look at the numbers.

For total cholesterol:
- Under 200 milligrams/deciliter (mg/dl) is desirable
- 200–239 mg/dl is borderline high risk
- 240 mg/dl or higher is high risk

For HDL (the "good" cholesterol):
- A level of 60 or higher offers some protection against heart disease

For LDL (the "bad" cholesterol):
- Optimal is less than 100 mg/dl
- Near or above optimal is 100–129 mg/dl
- Borderline high is 130–159 mg/dl
- High is 160–189 mg/dl
- Very high is 190 mg/dl or above

For triglycerides (the fat in your blood):
- Optimal is less than 100 mg/dl
- Normal is less than 150 mg/dl
- Borderline high is 150–199 mg/dl
- High is 200–499 mg/dl
- Very high is 500 mg/dl[3]

For blood pressure (guidelines from the American Heart Association):
- Normal is less than 120 systolic, less than 80 diastolic
- Prehypertension is 120–139 systolic, 80–89 diastolic
- Hypertension is 140 or higher systolic, 90 or higher diastolic[4]

For fasting blood glucose (taken after at least an eight-hour fast; guidelines from the American Diabetes Association):
- Normal fasting blood glucose should be below 100 mg/dl
- Prediabetes is a fasting blood glucose level between 100 and 125 mg/dl
- Diabetes is a fasting blood glucose level of 126 mg/dl or above[5]

DASH and the Prediabetes Diet Plan

After reading part 2 of this book, you're familiar with key tenets of the prediabetes diet plan: the importance of avoiding trans fats, limiting saturated fat (ideally less than 7 percent of your daily calories, or 16 grams a day for the average 2,000-calorie diet), and shifting to a more plant-based diet. Research suggests the most comprehensive and effective dietary approach to lowering your cardiovascular risk is to follow the DASH diet. DASH stands for "dietary approaches to stop hypertension," but it actually encompasses all the recommendations for a heart-healthy diet.[6] It's a comprehensive eating plan based on research funded by the National Heart, Lung, and Blood Institute. The institute found that taking on the DASH diet can reduce blood pressure in as little as two weeks. It incorporates a variety of dietary influences known to lower blood pressure: the diet is low in total fat, saturated fat, and cholesterol, and emphasizes fruits, vegetables, and fat-free or low-fat milk and milk products. It also includes whole grains, fish, poultry, and small portions of nuts, seeds, and legumes.

The DASH diet combination is rich in potassium, magnesium, calcium, lean protein, and fiber—all dietary elements known to keep blood pressure down. Most people are aware that sodium can also affect blood pressure. DASH recommends limiting sodium, both added at the table and in foods, to no more than 2,300 milligrams per day (the equivalent of 1 teaspoon), preferably even lower if possible, to around 1,500 milligrams per day. DASH is high-carb plan (about 55 percent of your daily calories), which is a little higher than recommended in the prediabetes

The DASH Diet (1,600 calories)

FOOD GROUP	SERVINGS PER DAY
Grains	6 servings
Vegetables	3 to 4 servings
Fruits	4 servings
Fat-free or 1 percent milk or milk products	2 to 3 servings
Lean meats, poultry, and fish	3 to 6 ounces
Nuts, seeds, and legumes	3 servings a week
Fats and oils	2 servings
Sweets and added sugars	0 (higher-calorie levels allow no more than 5 servings per week)

plan (I recommend somewhere around 45 percent of daily calories from carbs), but with a little attention to carb portions, the two plans can easily interface.

Looking at these DASH recommendations, you may be eating a little more lean protein (perhaps 6 to 8 ounces a day, or a little more if you are male or very physically active) and a little less carbohydrate, but that's okay. I'd suggest trimming the grain portions first and really emphasizing whole grains to get the benefit of the minerals and phytonutrients. Regarding prediabetes, you have the added concern of managing insulin resistance, which isn't good for your heart, so merging the best of both plans is the wisest approach. And don't forget exercise! It's one of the strongest lifestyle strategies there is for controlling both blood pressure and insulin resistance.

10

Exercise:
Time to Take It Seriously

Whether you love it, hate it, or fall somewhere in between, physical activity is an important part of a healthy lifestyle. This is particularly important if you have prediabetes because of the critical role exercise plays in weight management, insulin resistance, and cardiovascular risk. Research demonstrates that exercise is necessary for weight loss and particularly for weight-loss maintenance. Exercise acts as nature's insulin sensitizer by increasing the activity of glucose transporter 4 (GLUT 4), a protein that shuttles glucose out of the blood and into muscle and fat cells.[1] Exercise raises heart-healthy HDL cholesterol and lowers unhealthy LDL cholesterol and triglyceride levels. Exercise mobilizes belly fat, lowering the risk of diabetes and heart disease.[2] Regular exercise also lowers the risk of a number of cancers, Alzheimer's disease, depression, and anxiety. It also improves mood and helps people remain physically independent throughout their lives.[3]

Potent Medicine for Prediabetes

Many studies confirm that exercise improves insulin sensitivity in people with prediabetes, whether or not they lose weight along the way. In fact, in those with prediabetes, eating right and exercise may lower the risk of developing diabetes by an average of 50 percent![4] That is an enormous advantage regular exercisers have over more sedentary people. One recent study tried combining exercise with the diabetes drug metformin to see if this combination would even further improve insulin sensitivity (and in theory help avoid or slow the progression to type 2 diabetes) beyond either exercise or metformin alone. Subjects in the exercise groups exercised three times a week for sixty to seventy-five minutes over a twelve-week period, with two of the three sessions including strengthening exercise. Interestingly, researchers found an improvement in insulin sensitivity in all groups (exercising only, metformin only, and combination of metformin and exercise) that wasn't significantly different, providing some positive evidence for those people interested in avoiding diabetes *without* using medications.[5]

The catch is, you have to continue exercising to reap the benefits of exercise. One study of thirty-two women with polycystic ovary syndrome (PCOS), who are known to be at high risk for prediabetes, had them exercising regularly for three months; then half of the group continued to work out while the other half stopped exercising for another twelve weeks. Both groups showed improvement in their body mass index (BMI), insulin resistance, cholesterol levels, and measures of fitness after the first twelve weeks, but after twenty-four weeks the exercising group continued to improve (in all of those measures) while those who stopped exercising showed worsening of these parameters.[6] The National Weight Control Registry participants exercise about sixty minutes a day to maintain their weight loss. Independent of weight loss, however, exercise improves cardiovascular fitness, lowers blood pressure, trims belly fat, and improves mood.[7]

Experts Weigh In on Activity

Despite the many benefits of exercise, surveys over the past decade show that Americans haven't gotten much better at getting off the couch. The American College of Sports Medicine (ACSM) has long been sounding the alarm about the hazards of a sedentary lifestyle, and in 2007 the ACSM issued some very reasonable recommendations for activity to improve health and quality of life. These guidelines are as follows: moderately intense cardio thirty minutes a day, five days a week (or vigorously intense cardio twenty minutes a day, three days a week), and eight to ten strength-training exercises, with eight to twelve repetitions of each exercise, twice a week.

The thirty-minute recommendation is to maintain health and lower the risk of disease, but to lose weight and keep it off, ACSM notes exercisers need sixty to ninety minutes of physical activity at least five days a week.[8]

In 2008 the US Department of Health and Human Services (HHS) also got more aggressive with its exercise recommendations, issuing the first ever Physical Activity Guidelines for Americans, which outlined exactly how much activity, and what kinds, are needed to help Americans control their weight and reduce their risk of some of the country's major health threats.[9] Thousands of studies have affirmed the benefits of physical activity for people of all ages and abilities, with very little risk. Recommendations were made for three age groups: children and adolescents, adults (including pregnant women and those with disabilities), and older adults. Daily life activity varies widely among individuals, so the recommendations focus on activities that, when added to light day-to-day activities, improve health. Examples of health-enhancing activities are brisk walking, jogging, swimming, dancing, lifting weights, and yoga. To help people rate their personal activity level, an advisory committee identified four levels:

- Inactive (no activity beyond baseline daily activities)
- Low (beyond baseline but fewer than 150 minutes per week)
- Medium (150–300 minutes per week)
- High (more than 300 minutes per week)

Research suggests that the sweet spot for receiving consistent benefits from activity is an accumulated minimum of 150 minutes per week of moderate-intensity aerobic activities, such as walking briskly, water aerobics, ballroom and line dancing, biking on level ground or with few hills, canoeing, general gardening (raking, trimming shrubs), sports where you catch and throw (baseball, softball, volleyball), and tennis (doubles). Or you can step it up and get the same benefits from seventy-five minutes per week of vigorous-intensity activity, like aerobic dance (includes recreational dancing), biking faster than ten miles an hour, heavy gardening (digging, hoeing), hiking uphill, jumping rope, martial arts (karate), sports with a lot of running (basketball, hockey, soccer), swimming fast or swimming laps, tennis (singles), and race walking, jogging, or running.

Exercise more than this and it's a bonus, as health continues to improve as activity increases. If the thought of exercising makes you groan, keep in mind that as little as ten minutes of activity counts toward improving your health. These guidelines also encourage muscle-strengthening activities two or more days a week to increase and preserve bone and muscle strength. Strengthening activities include weight training, resistance bands, weight-bearing calisthenics, and heavy gardening. Beyond its stress management and flexibility benefits, forms of yoga that are weight-bearing are also considered strengthening exercise. For many people, losing weight and keeping it off will require 300 minutes or more of moderate activity per week (that's 60 minutes a day, five days a week), or 150 minutes of vigorous activity. Most people also need to make a conscious effort to eat less when they start exercising since there's a natural tendency to eat more, because either you're more hungry or you think you've "earned" an extra treat because you've worked out.

Accruing Your Minutes

Now that you know your numbers, how can you piece together enough exercise? Check out these ways to rack up the recommended amount of activity.

For 150 minutes a week of moderate activity:

- Thirty minutes of brisk walking (moderate intensity) five days a week; resistance bands (strengthening) two days a week
- Twenty-five minutes of jogging (vigorous intensity) three days a week; weightlifting two days a week
- Thirty minutes of stationary bike or elliptical two days a week; sixty minutes of dancing one evening; thirty minutes of lawn mowing one afternoon; heavy gardening (strengthening) on two days
- Forty-five minutes of tennis doubles (moderate intensity) on two days; thirty minutes of brisk walking on two days; weight machines (strengthening) two days a week

For 75 minutes a week of vigorous activity:

- Thirty minutes of aerobic dancing two days a week; fifteen minutes swimming laps one day; weightlifting two days a week
- Thirty minutes of fast bicycling two days a week; fifteen minutes of jogging one day; weight machines two days a week

For 300 minutes a week of moderate activity:

- Forty-five minutes of brisk walking daily; resistance bands two days a week
- Sixty minutes of doubles tennis two days a week; sixty minutes of brisk walking three days a week; weight machines on two days
- Forty-five minutes of stationary cycling two days a week; forty-five minutes of water aerobics on one day, thirty minutes of outdoor cycling two days a week; sixty minutes of general gardening on one day; thirty minutes of brisk walking two days a week; resistance bands two days a week

For 150 minutes a week of vigorous activity:

- Sixty minutes of aerobic dancing two days a week; thirty minutes of singles tennis one day a week; weight machines on two days
- Forty-five minutes of jogging two days a week; sixty minutes of hiking one day a week; weight-bearing calisthenics two days a week

Determining Your Exercise Intensity

How hard should you push yourself, and how do you determine the exercise intensity? The HHS guidelines offer these helpful hints: When exercising moderately, you should be able to talk but not sing. During vigorous activity, you shouldn't be able to say more than a few words before breathing heavily. You can trade off minutes by substituting one minute of vigorous activity for two minutes of moderate activity. For example, fifteen minutes of jogging and fifteen minutes of brisk walking is equal to forty-five minutes of brisk walking alone.

Other Benefits of Exercise

The Physical Activity Guidelines for Americans cite many additional benefits of exercise beyond improving your health. Quality-of-life reasons to increase your activity include lower rates of depression, more fun in your life, enjoyment of the outdoors, and improved body image. The guidelines also conclude that for the vast majority of people, the benefits of exercise far outweigh any risk—particularly if activities are varied to avoid overuse injuries—but people with concerns should check with their doctor first.

If your budget allows, consider signing on with a personal trainer. People tend to make greater gains working with a trainer and may be more likely to stick with their programs. Finding an exercise buddy—maybe a spouse, coworker, friend, or family member—also increases your odds of setting an exercise plan and sticking with it.

Part 4

FINE-TUNING THE PREDIABETES DIET PLAN

11

Sensible Supplementation

Like most nutritionists, I prefer a food-first approach to meeting nutrient needs. Research has demonstrated that popping a few vitamin pills won't compensate for a lousy diet, but there is some sensible supplementation that most people might benefit from, whether or not they have prediabetes. When I consider which supplements make sense for people with prediabetes or insulin resistance, I draw on what is known about genetics and how historically humans have eaten. For example, we were genetically designed to run around naked, being exposed to the sun for much of the day, giving us ample opportunity for skin and sun exposure to synthesize "the sunshine vitamin"—vitamin D. Most of us could use more of it today. And in order to accumulate enough carbohydrates, proteins, and fats (and therefore calories) to survive, humans had to hunt and gather many different foods, each with their own unique balance of vitamins, minerals, phytonutrients, and omega-3 fats. As a result, the caveman's diet may have been a lot more nutritionally diverse than the average American's diet today. People can be more selective today, and some people end up eating many of the same foods most days. Dietary supplements can help pick up the slack for what we should be getting but often aren't getting enough of. There are some interesting suggestions of dietary supplements and herbs to help manage insulin resistance, with varying degrees of scientific backing. Because the goal of this book is to provide advice on the most studied aspects of diet and lifestyle in managing prediabetes and preventing diabetes, I won't delve into herbs and alternative therapies here. I have enough respect for the potentially medicinal effects of herbs to avoid dabbling in a field that is not my area of expertise.

The Basic Multivitamin

A basic multivitamin provides around 100 percent of the daily values (DV), the amounts recommended per day for a variety of vitamins and minerals. Most multis contain around 100 percent (sometimes a bit more) for the vitamins, but smaller amounts of the minerals. Some minerals are bulky, so you wouldn't be able to fit a day's worth in a pill without making it prohibitively huge. Multis often contain only about 160 milligrams or so of calcium, for example, though women's multis may provideup to 500 milligrams of supplemental calcium. For some minerals there is no established recommended dietary allowance, so no percent DV will appear.

The main argument in favor of taking a multivitamin/multimineral supplement is that most people don't eat perfect diets every day, so it gives you a little added assurance. Very few people get enough vitamin D, so some basic supplementation is warranted. metformin, a medication commonly used to treat prediabetes and diabetes, can interfere with vitamin B_{12} absorption over time, so a little extra is a good idea. If you think your diet is pretty well balanced, by all means skip the multi and just take vitamin D and a B_{12} supplement if you're on metformin. Like almost all dietary supplements, multivitamin/multimineral supplements should be taken with food to help with absorption and avoid risk of stomach upset.

Magnesium and Insulin Resistance

Multis may include some magnesium, although generally only about 25 percent of the DV. Magnesium plays a role in blood sugar regulation (crucial to the function of insulin), and studies have found that higher dietary magnesium intake is associated with lower fasting insulin concentrations and a reduced risk of developing type 2 diabetes.[1] The recommended dietary allowance for magnesium is 420 milligrams for men and 320 milligrams for women over age thirty.[2] Magnesium status tends to reflect the overall quality of the diet, so your best bet is to eat more high-magnesium foods. These include whole grain breads and cereals, brown rice, wheat germ, nuts, beans, spinach, artichokes, and avocados. If you decide to supplement, however, keep your dose well below the safe upper limit of 350 milligrams per day. The recommended daily allowances above for men and women are based on intake of magnesium from food, and don't present a problem because your body eliminates what it doesn't need.

Too much magnesium taken all at once in pill form can cause diarrhea and abdominal pain.[3]

Vitamin D and Prediabetes

Research suggests that many Americans may have inadequate blood levels of vitamin D, defined as less than 30 nanograms per milliliter).[4] According to research published in *Nutrition Journal*, low levels of vitamin D are believed to be associated with higher rates of illness and death from a host of health problems, including bone disease, diabetes, cardiovascular disease, cancer, autoimmune diseases, mood disorders, and possibly other conditions.[5] Vitamin D deficiency is common because we're genetically designed to synthesize vitamin D from sun exposure (rather than eating it). Food sources of vitamin D include fish, oysters, cheese, and egg yolks as well as fortified foods such as milk and some juices and yogurts. The reality is, however, you'd have to eat a lot of these foods to get even the current recommendation of 600 IUs per day (800 IUs for those over age seventy). Some vitamin D experts have deemed even these levels too low. Many experts recommend 800 to 1,000 IUs of vitamin D per day for everyone who isn't regularly exposed to the sun.[6]

Vitamin D deficiency has been proposed by some to be a risk factor in the development of insulin resistance and type 2 diabetes by affecting either insulin sensitivity or pancreatic cell function, or both. The prevalence of type 2 diabetes seems to be higher in those who are vitamin D deficient.[7] Beyond diabetes prevention, there are loads of reasons to avoid deficiency, so it's reasonable to aim for a total vitamin D intake of 800 to 1,000 IUs from all supplement sources (calcium often contains vitamin D as well). Vitamin D_3, or cholecalciferol, may offer a leg up in repleting vitamin D levels, so look for this form in over-the-counter supplements. After two or three months, you can have your vitamin D level checked to see if this dose is adequate. The test is called 25-hydroxyvitamin D, and as mentioned earlier the desirable blood level is 30 ng/ml or higher. Many people have very low vitamin D levels (below 20 ng/ml), which will need to be replaced with a large amount of vitamin D up front—often a prescription dose of 50,000 IUs of vitamin D_2 once a week for eight weeks—to initially ramp up vitamin D levels. After this time, people may be able to settle into a maintenance dose of 1,000 to 2,000 IUs of vitamin D_3 per day.

Omega-3 Fats: Eat More Fish or Supplement

In recent years the scientific evidence supporting the importance of omega-3 fats to overall health has skyrocketed. The science for loading up on omega-3s is strongest for managing a number of cardiovascular risk factors. Omega-3s have been found to lower blood triglyceride levels and blood pressure, and may slow the accumulation of cholesterol plaques in the arteries—all of which may reduce the risk of heart attack and stroke. Research has been mixed (and is ongoing) but suggests that omega-3s may be helpful in improving insulin resistance by countering the inflammation associated with IR and possibly helping to slow the progression of pre-diabetes to diabetes in other ways.[8]

The three major types of omega-3 fatty acids are DHA (docosa-hexaenoic acid), EPA (eicosapentaenoic acid), and ALA (alpha-linolenic acid). ALA is found in seeds; canola, flaxseed, and soybean oils; green leafy vegetables; nuts; and beans. DHA and EPA are found in fatty fish like salmon, mackerel, herring, lake trout, sardines, and tuna as well as in fish oil supplements. To cover your bases, aim to include both fish and plant sources of omega-3s in your diet. DHA and EPA are the long-chain omega-3s found in fish and fish oil, and are considered more physiologically active in the body. ALA is a short-chain omega-3, which needs to be converted to either DHA or EPA to be used most efficiently. Unfortunately, the body converts very little ALA to EPA or DHA, but ALA has unique benefits of its own, so it's best to consume both. If you opt for supplements, choose a brand that provides at least 600 to 700 milligrams or more of total omega-3s (DHA and EPA) per dose.

Other Supplements for Prediabetes

Some supplements are marketed to people with prediabetes, including those that target insulin resistance. By no means should you feel compelled to take these, but you may read about them and want to know the state of the science.

Chromium picolinate. Chromium is a trace mineral (needed in small amounts) that plays a role in glucose regulation by sensitizing cells to the action of insulin and possibly increasing cell insulin receptor number and activity. Some evidence shows that taking chromium picolinate supplements (the most common oral form) may help lower fasting blood glucose, insulin, and hemoglobin A1C levels, and increase insulin sensitivity in people with type 2 diabetes. Not all research supports these benefits, however. Food sources of chromium include onions, tomatoes, oysters, whole grains, bran cereals, and potatoes.[9] Brewer's yeast is also a good dietary source of chromium, although not an easy supplement for some people to stomach.

It is estimated that women need about 20 to 25 micrograms of chromium per day and men 30 to 35 micrograms per day, depending on age.[10] Although there is no safe upper limit set for chromium supplements, the National Academy of Sciences has established a "safe and adequate daily dietary intake" range for chromium of 50 to 200 micrograms per day, so if you decide to give it a try, you may want to limit it to no more than 200 micrograms.[11] As chromium could affect your insulin metabolism, talk to your doctor first before taking it with metformin or any other diabetes medicine. For those on thyroid medication, chromium picolinate may bind with levothyroxine (Synthroid), so be sure to take the medication and the supplement at least three to four hours apart. Because of lack of safety data, chromium supplements should be avoided by pregnant women or those who could become pregnant.

Cinnamon. This widely used spice may help lower blood glucose levels. Research has been mixed and inconclusive, and it could be that very high doses, or specific cinnamon extracts, may be needed to produce any benefit.[12] Until more is known about this spice and glucose levels, enjoy cinnamon for its great taste and continue to focus on diet, exercise, and your new healthy lifestyle.

Choosing a Quality Supplement

Unlike pharmaceutical drugs, where production is overseen by the US Food and Drug Administration, quality standards for production of dietary supplements in this country are largely voluntary. Under the law, dietary supplement manufacturers are supposed to make sure their products are safe before they go to market and that the claims on their labels are accurate and truthful. Supplements are not reviewed by the government before they're sold, however, and there have been instances where the government has stepped in and removed harmful products from the market. Here are a few things to consider when selecting a supplement:

- Is it made by a large dietary supplement or pharmaceutical company? Large companies are more likely to have stringent internal production standards.
- Does it have a "USP Verified" mark on the label? The USP Dietary Supplement Verification Program is a voluntary testing and auditing program that verifies the quality, purity, and potency of dietary supplements.
- Make note of the serving size on the label so you know how many pills you'll have to take to get the dose of nutrients listed on the label.

Above all, know what you're taking and why! I'm amazed at the number of clients I see who have no idea why they're taking a certain supplement. It's a good idea to periodically review your supplements with a health professional because sometimes recommendations change.

12

Mastering the Market: An Aisle-by-Aisle Shopping Guide

Wouldn't you like to sit down most nights to a meal that tastes good and is good for you? If so, you need to take control of your food environment. Populate your home and workplace with things you should be eating, and make it difficult to access foods you may have trouble limiting. It's not about totally depriving yourself of foods you love. If you want an ice cream, go out and get a child-sized cone—you just don't need a half gallon in your freezer tempting you every night. Want to save calories—and money? Pack a lunch from home and make it the night before so you don't run out of time to make it in the morning. Too tempted when you walk into the grocery store? Consider an online grocery shopping service like Peapod, Wal-Mart, or Netgrocer.com.

Taking control of your food environment requires planning, a big part of which starts in the grocery store. Let's take a look at how to make good choices in the market.

Reading Food Labels

The shopping lists in this chapter are organized by food category and begin with a brief description of what to look for on the label. Brand-name foods that meet the criteria are listed, but it's important to be able to navigate a food label yourself in case you find something that looks appealing and you want to know if it's a good choice. Pay attention to several key things on the Nutrition Facts label.

Nutrition Facts

Serving Size 1 slice
Servings Per Container 20

Amount Per Serving

Calories 90	Calories from Fat 15

	% Daily Value*
Total Fat 2g	3%
Saturated Fat 0g	0%
Trans Fat 0g	
Cholesterol 0mg	0%
Sodium 130mg	5%
Total Carbohydrate 15g	5%
Dietary Fiber 2g	8%
Sugars 1g	
Protein 4g	

Vitamin A 0%	Vitamin C 0%
Calcium 4%	Iron 4%

Percent daily value reflects "as packaged" food.

* Percent daily values are based on a 2,000 calorie diet. Your daily values may be higher or lower depending on your calorie needs:

	Calories:	2,000	2,500
Total Fat	Less than	65g	80g
Sat Fat	Less than	20g	25g
Cholesterol	Less than	300mg	300mg
Sodium	Less than	2,400mg	2,400mg
Total Carbohydrate		300g	375g
Dietary Fiber		25g	30g
Calories per gram:	Fat 9	Carbohydrate 4	Protein 4

Serving size. The most important element on the food label is the serving size because everything else you subsequently read is based on that portion. If the label portion is ½ cup and your portion is 1 cup, you need to double everything on the label. That's twice as many calories, fat grams, and carbs.

Calories and calories from fat. This information is helpful if you're trying to determine the percentage of calories from fat. For example, if your goal is to get 30 percent of your total calories from fat, and the fat calories on the label are a third or less of the total calories, then the food item may be a good choice (getting roughly 30 percent or less of its calories from fat).

Total fat. This number helps you determine if the food is "low fat"—which means 3 grams of fat or less per serving. Not all foods need to fit this definition, but it gives you a reference point: something with 5 grams of fat per serving is pretty close to low fat, 8 grams per serving is getting up there, and 16 grams of fat in one hot dog is a lot!

Saturated fat and trans fats. These should be limited as much as possible in your diet, so ideally these two numbers should be zero. "Low saturated" means no more than 1 gram of saturated fat per serving, so aim for that with as many food choices as possible. Any amount of trans fat is considered unhealthy, so stick to that goal of zero. If a nutrient is present in less than 0.5 grams per serving, the manufacturer is allowed to round down to zero on the label. This means there could be a hair less than 0.5 gram of trans fat per serving that could add up if you eat two or three servings. To play it safe, avoid foods with "shortening," "hydrogenated," or "partially hydrogenated" fat listed as an ingredient—these are the main sources of trans fats in the diet.

Cholesterol. "Low cholesterol" means no more than 20 milligrams per serving and should be limited to 300 milligrams per day.

Sodium. "Low sodium" means less than 140 milligrams per serving and should be limited to 2,400 milligrams per day (2,300 milligrams if you're following the DASH diet).

Total carbohydrates. These are of key interest for anyone managing prediabetes. As you now know, a carbohydrate choice is a portion that contains 15 grams of carb, so the total carb number should be divided by 15 to see roughly how many carb choices are in a serving of the food. In the example label on the preceding page, the 15 grams of carb per serving of this food is one carb choice. If the total carbs were 40 grams, it would be roughly two-and-a-half servings. Estimating is good enough.

Dietary fiber. This is another very important number for the prediabetes diet plan. The more you eat the better. A "high-fiber" food means there are 5 grams or more per serving. A food that is considered a "good source" of fiber has 2.5 grams to 4.9 grams per serving. Remember, with any food that contains 5 grams of fiber or more per serving, the American Diabetes Association says you are allowed to subtract half the grams of fiber from the total carbs in your carb count. I'm assuming that if you're reading this book, you are not diabetic, so it's okay to subtract any fiber grams from the total carbohydrate number. The incentive for choosing higher-fiber foods is that you get to subtract more carb grams!

Sugar. There is currently no official definition for "low sugar" because food labels don't differentiate between natural sugars (fructose from fruit and lactose from milk) and added sweeteners. "Reduced sugar" means 25 percent less sugar than the original food item, which doesn't necessarily mean much if the original is loaded with sugar. A reasonable number to aim for is around 8 grams of sugar or less per serving.

Protein. The presence of protein in a carb-containing food helps you feel fuller longer and slows the digestion of carbs to blood glucose.

Percent daily value. This is the amount of a nutrient that will be satisfied by eating a serving of the food. The percentages are based on the levels of nutrients recommended as part of a healthy 2,000-calorie diet as listed at the bottom of the Nutrition Facts label. For example, a serving of our sample food uses up 5 percent of the saturated fat allowance for the day (listed at the bottom of the label as 20 grams). These percentages are also provided for some vitamins and minerals. It's worth noting that the calcium percentage is based on the DV of 1,000 milligrams, so if you replace the percentage sign with a "0," that's your milligrams. In our example, the 4 percent DV of calcium represents 40 milligrams of calcium.[1]

Shopping for Plant Foods

When buying produce, stock up on both fresh and frozen vegetables (so you have a backup plan when you've run out of fresh veggies). I'm a huge fan of steam-ready microwavable vegetables that are steamed right in the bag like microwave popcorn. According to the food companies, all the plastics used are FDA-approved as microwave safe. For those who prefer to avoid cooking in plastic, steam fresh or frozen veggies in an inexpensive stainless-steel steamer or microwave in a glass dish. Frozen fruits are also nice to have on hand to mix with yogurt (thaw slightly first) or blend into a smoothie.

A critical component of the prediabetes diet plan is to eat more plant foods. Stretch beyond your old standbys when shopping and resolve to include more color in your diet:

- **Blue/purple.** Blueberries, blackberries, eggplant, figs, plums, prunes, purple cabbage, and purple grapes.

- **Green.** Artichokes, arugula, asparagus, avocado, bok choy, broccoli, broccoli rabe, brussels sprouts, cabbage, celery, cucumbers, endive, greens, green apples, green beans, green grapes, green olives, green peppers, honeydew melon, kiwi, limes, lettuce, okra, peas, snow peas, spinach, and zucchini.
- **Orange/yellow.** Apricots, winter squash, cantaloupe, carrots, grapefruit, yellow beets, lemons, mangoes, nectarines, oranges, papaya, peaches, yellow pears, pineapples, pumpkin, sweet potato, tangerines, yams, corn, and summer squash.
- **Red.** Red apples, beets, cherries, cranberries, pink grapefruit, pomegranates, raspberries, red grapes, red peppers, radishes, radicchio, red onions, strawberries, tomatoes, and watermelon.
- **White/gold.** Cauliflower, garlic, jicama, mushrooms, onions, parsnips, potatoes, shallots, turnips, and bosc pears.

Starter Shopping List

Now that you know how to read labels, let's create a shopping list to help guide you through the aisles at the supermarket. This list is by no means all-inclusive. Criteria are provided at the top of each category that you can apply to anything of interest. Examples of foods that meet the criteria are here to get you started. So start experimenting and see what you can add to—or should subtract from—your kitchen.

Poultry. Note that "cold cuts" are elsewhere, later in the list.
- Fresh chicken breast: buy in bulk when on sale and freeze individual portions in freezer bags
- Frozen chicken breast: available in large zip-lock bags as breast or tenders, or individually frozen in plastic
- Chicken legs and thighs: buy fresh or frozen, without the skin to trim fat calories
- Precooked chicken pieces: beware the sodium in flavored varieties
- Canned chicken: use for sandwiches and salads
- Limit chicken wings, chicken nuggets, and any other breaded chicken product to only occasional use because of high fat and salt content
- Fresh or frozen turkey breast
- Ground turkey: buy only 90 percent lean or leaner

Seafood. Buy fresh, frozen, or canned depending on use.
- Any kind of fish, shrimp, and other shellfish that's not fried
- Canned tuna, salmon, or shrimp
- Salmon lox
- Smoked salmon

Meat. Look for the words "loin," "round," "flank," "chuck" or "90 percent lean" or leaner; limit yourself to no more than 18 ounces of animal protein a week.[2]
- Beef: eye of the round, top round steak, top round roast, sirloin steak, top loin steak, tenderloin steak, flank steak, and chuck arm pot roast
- Veal: cutlet, blade or arm steak, rib roast, and rib or loin chop
- Pork: tenderloin, top loin roast, top loin chop, center loin chop, sirloin roast, loin rib chop, and shoulder blade steak
- Lamb: leg, loin chop, and arm chop

Miscellaneous protein. These are great protein choices for anyone—not just vegetarians.
- Eggs and egg substitutes
- Soy foods: tofu, tempeh, edamame, and TVP (textured vegetable protein)
- Beans (chickpeas, kidney beans, and so on) and peas
- Veggie burgers
- Hummus
- Quinoa

Fats and oils. Focus on heart-healthy fats, but remember that all fats are equal in calories no matter how heart healthy they are.
- Olive, canola, or peanut oil
- Tub spreads: trans fat–free, such as Olivio, Smart Balance, Brummel & Brown, Promise, many "light" spreads
- Light mayonnaise
- Low-fat salad dressings (these generally taste better than fat-free, but watch portions)
- Olives
- Avocado and guacamole

- Nuts, seeds, and nut butters (there is no need to buy reduced-fat peanut butter—the real thing has the same calories and tastes much better, although do watch your portions)

Cereals. Look for cereals with at least 3 grams, preferably 5 grams or more, of fiber and no more than 8 grams of sugar per serving. If your favorite cereal is higher in sugar, try mixing ¼ cup of it with ¾ cup low-sugar, high-fiber flakes.

- General Mills cereals: Fiber One, Total Whole Grain, Wheaties, Wheat and Multibran Chex, Multigrain Cheerios (other flavored versions of Cheerios, including Honey Nut, Apple, and Berry, have only 2 grams of fiber per serving)
- Kellogg's cereals: Complete Oat Bran and Wheat Bran Flakes, Kellogg's All Bran, Kellogg's Special K Protein Plus
- Post cereals: Shredded Wheat, Shredded Wheat and Bran, Bran Flakes, 100 percent Bran, Post Grape Nut Flakes
- Quaker cereals: Corn Bran, Oatmeal
- Barbara's cereals: Original Puffins, Cinnamon Puffins (not Peanut Butter Puffs), Shredded Wheat, Multigrain Shredded Spoonfuls
- Health Valley or Nature's Path cereals: Any of their whole grain flakes
- Kashi cereals: GoLean, Heart to Heart, 7 Whole Grain Flakes, Autumn Wheat Mini Wheats, any others with at least 3 grams of fiber and roughly 3 grams of fat and 8 grams of sugar or less per serving
- Cascadian Farm cereals: Multigrain Squares, Purely O's, any others with at least 3 grams of fiber and roughly 3 grams of fat and 8 grams of sugar or less per serving
- Trader Joe's and Whole Foods stores carry many varieties of cereal that meet these criteria; read the labels.

Crackers. Look for low-fat crackers (no more than 3 grams of fat), 2 grams of fiber or more, and no trans fats.

- Kashi TLC Honey Sesame, Natural Ranch, and Original 7 Grain
- Wheat Thins: Reduced Fat, Fiber Selects
- Triscuits: Reduced Fat, Thin Crisps, and Minis
- Ak-Mak 100% Whole Wheat

- Wasa Multigrain
- Kavli Crispbread
- Graham crackers (any brand)

Bread products. Breads, bagels, English muffins, and other bread products should have the word "whole" in the first ingredient (as in "whole wheat," "whole grain," and "whole oat") and contain at least 2 to 3 grams of fiber per slice. Choose those with calories as close as possible to 70 to 90 calories per slice.

- Freihofer's Stone Ground 100% Whole Wheat
- Wonder Stone Ground 100% Whole Wheat
- Weight Watchers 100% Whole Wheat Bread and English Muffins
- Arnold Health-full 10 Grain; 100% Whole Wheat or Multigrain Sandwich Thins; 100% Whole Wheat Sandwich Rolls
- Pepperidge Farm Carb Style 100% Whole Wheat, 7 Grain, Light Style Extra Fiber, Soft Wheat, and 100% Whole Wheat Cinnamon Raisin
- Bagels: Whole grain mini bagels, Thomas's 100% Whole Wheat Bagel Thins or English Muffins

Cold cuts. Look for low-fat varieties (3 grams of fat per serving); some are available in low-sodium versions.

- Sliced ham
- Sliced turkey
- Sliced chicken
- Lean roast beef

Cheeses. Look for cheeses with 5 grams of fat or less per ounce or slice. These will be made with fat-free, low-fat, or part-skim milk. Some cheeses below have slightly more fat but are still good choices if eaten in moderation.

- String cheese: part-skim mozzarella
- Laughing Cow Light Creamy Swiss Original
- Jarlsberg light
- Sargento reduced-fat deli-style thin
- Kraft 2 percent milk Deli Deluxe

- Cabot 50 percent reduced-fat cheddar
- Cracker Barrel 2 percent milk (6 grams of fat)
- Laughing Cow Mini Babybel Mild
- Sargento reduced-fat sharp cheddar sticks
- American: Smart Beat, Kraft-free singles, Borden fat-free singles, Kraft 2% milk singles, Land-O-Lake reduced-fat or low-fat
- Alpine Lace reduced-fat cheese
- Feta: President fat-free feta, Stella feta, Athenos reduced-fat feta

Yogurts. Unless it's plain (unflavored), yogurt may contain large amounts of added sugar unless marked "light," which means it's been artificially sweetened. Look for those with 20 grams of total carbs or less per 6 ounces (usually the case with Greek yogurts). Greek yogurts have two to three times the protein of regular yogurts.

- Stonyfield Farm: plain or flavored
- Dannon Light & Fit or fat-free plain yogurt
- Yoplait Light
- Greek style: Chobani nonfat Greek yogurt, Fage nonfat Greek yogurt, Dannon Light & Fit Greek Yogurt, Activia Greek 4-ounce yogurts
- Other 1 percent or nonfat Greek yogurts

Milk. Milk should be skim or 1 percent milkfat.

- Garelick Over-the-Moon: 1 percent fat or fat-free (both have the taste of whole milk)
- Simply Smart: nonfat milk with the taste of 2 percent milk
- Silk unflavored or light soy milk
- Silk soy milk (enhanced) with 35 percent recommended daily value for calcium
- 8th Continent soy milk
- Almond milk (check flavored varieties for added sugars; very low in protein with the exception of So Delicious Almond Plus, which has 5 grams of protein per 8 ounces)

Beverages. All beverages should be calorie-free or have no more than 40 calories per 8 ounces.

- Water
- Diet V-8 Splash
- Light Ocean Spray cranberry juice and blends
- Minute Maid Light juice beverages
- Vitamin Water Zero
- Sobe Life Waters
- Diet iced teas
- Fruit2O
- Crystal Light
- All diet sodas and seltzer waters

Frozen foods. Some frozen foods may be low in calories and fat, but many are still very high in sodium. Look for frozen dinners with 45 to 60 grams of carb, at least 14 to 20 grams of protein, no more than 8 to 10 grams of fat, and no more than 500 milligrams of sodium. Add extra fresh or frozen vegetables and fruits to boost the plant content of the meal.

- Frozen meals: Natural food stores (or sections in the supermarket) usually offer healthier frozen dinners (Amy's, Organic Bistro, and Kashi are some good brands).
- Vegetarian alternatives: Gardenburgers (meatless, soy-based); Boca products (meatless, soy-based), including burgers, chicken patties, meatless chili, breakfast patties; Morning Star Farms veggie products, including "sausage" links and patties, soy "crumbles" for recipes

Snack foods. Look for low-fat options, meaning 3 grams of fat or less per serving with zero trans fats. Many snack foods are carbs that should be paired with protein for a more filling snack.

- Pretzels: any brands except for those flavored with fat
- Popcorn: light and low-fat varieties
- Potato and tortilla chips: baked and "crisps" varieties
- Breadsticks
- Corn or rice cakes: plain or flavored

- Crunchy granola bars or chewy varieties with at least 3 grams of fiber and less than 150 calories per bar
- Pudding: low-fat and sugar-free varieties
- Cookies: limit to one serving of trans fat–free cookies to control calories. Remember to factor in the carbs. If you can't limit them, don't buy them!
- Low-fat frozen desserts: preferably sugar-free. Limit to one serving to control calories. Remember to factor in the carbs. Skinny Cow ice cream sandwiches, Welch's No Sugar Added Fruit Juice Bars, Edy's Carb Smart Fudge Bars, Klondike Slim Bear Bars (no sugar added)

13

Considerations When Dining Out

It may be healthier to plan and prepare a homemade meal every night, but in today's on-the-go society that's not always possible. Eating out can be a challenge: we are hardwired to overeat in the presence of large portions—particularly when the food is infused with fat, salt, and sugar. Part of the reason it's so hard to resist overeating when dining out is that many of us still experience that "yippee!" feeling we may have developed back when we were kids and eating out was a special treat. If you rarely dine out, what you order doesn't matter as much. The occasional splurge will easily be offset by your eating well most days (remember the 80/20 rule).

But Americans have become accustomed to eating out more often, and restaurants have sought to cater to every taste and price point. Some restaurants make it easier than others for you to make decent choices, but often the portions are too big even if the choice is healthy. Fast-food restaurants make it nearly impossible to make a decent choice unless you order a kid's meal, which technically should be enough for the average adult as well. Chain restaurants such as TGI Fridays, Applebee's, Chili's, and the Cheesecake Factory may offer a "weight watchers" item, but the rest of the menu is loaded with highly processed, tough-to-resist foods that are high in fat, salt, and sugar delivered in enormous portions containing twice as many calories as you think.

A smarter bet is to dine at smaller restaurants where the food is prepared on-site and you can get an idea of what's actually in your dish. No matter where you're eating out, the restaurant-sized portion is probably at least 30 to 50 percent larger than what you should be having (unless you're a marathon runner!). The amount of fat, salt, and sugar in the meal is also probably a lot higher than you think. If you're really determined to eat a healthy meal, request substitutions (an extra vegetable instead of french fries, for example) and modifications (sauce on the side, less butter). With the rising rates of food allergies in this country and our increasing focus on health, many restaurants are used to being asked what's in their food and if something can be served differently. No matter what you order, portion control is key. Use these strategies to deal with the often difficult reality of dining out:

- Split a large entrée with someone and pair it with a side salad.
- Ask the server to pack half your entrée in a take-home container before you're served.
- Look for "lighter-fare" items on the menu that are smaller portions or made with lower-calorie ingredients.
- Avoid all-you-can-eat buffets! Few of us can resist the temptation to overeat in this setting.

Navigating the Menu

Learning how to spot healthier options on the menu is critical, particularly if you travel for work and eat out a lot. Try using the website www.healthydiningfinder.com before a trip: simply plug in the zip code you're traveling to and see what restaurants offer healthy choices in the area. Search results include the nutritional breakdown for the items offered. If you're not sure how a certain dish is prepared, be sure to ask your server. Knowledge is power when making smarter, healthier choices in restaurants. Certain words or phrases on the menu imply some cooking methods that are healthier than others. Use these guidelines for ordering.

Meat and poultry. When ordering meat and poultry, avoid items that are "fried," "crispy," "pan-fried," "sautéed," "stuffed," or prepared "parmigiana-style." These methods are generally high in fat and calories. Instead, look for these words on the menu that suggest a lighter style of cooking: "steamed," "broiled," "baked," "grilled," "poached," and "roasted." Fatty cuts of meat include rib eye, porterhouse, and T-bone. Leaner cuts are London broil, filet mignon, round or flank steak, sirloin tip, and tenderloin. Request that visible fat be removed from meat and skin be removed from poultry before it's served. Request that gravies, sauces, and dressings be served on the side (and don't use it all!). This way you can control how much you eat or skip it completely.

Vegetables. High-fat vegetable dishes to avoid are anything described on the menu as "fried," "scalloped," "au gratin," served in a cream or cheese sauce, or tempura-style (fried vegetables). Remembering the balanced-plate approach, choose entrées with a lot of vegetables. Cover half your plate with vegetables by trading in the starch choice for a second vegetable. You can then savor a roll with a pat of butter as your starch. Look for plain vegetable choices described as "steamed," "grilled," or "roasted." Request a lemon wedge or vinegar to add flavor.

Starchy sides. High-fat starchy side dishes may be described as "fried," "scalloped," "au gratin," or served in a cream or cheese sauce. Although they might be tough to find in some restaurants, when possible order whole grains such as brown or wild rice, whole wheat tortillas, and whole wheat pasta. Higher-fat starch choices include rice pilaf, stuffed or twice-baked potatoes, and vegetable or potato casseroles. A reasonable portion of plain rice or half a baked potato are better options. A teaspoon of butter melted over the top adds 40 calories, and two tablespoons of sour cream add 50 calories.

Salad. To avoid overeating on the main entrée, enjoy a premeal salad with low-fat dressing (a low-fat vinaigrette rather than a creamy dressing is best). To conserve calories, ask for dressing on the side and dip your fork into it before grabbing a bite of salad. But be smart about your choices and pay attention to the ingredients. Salad bar add-ons like mayonnaise-based pasta and potato salads, oil-based marinated vegetable or bean salads, cheeses, croutons, and bacon bits can undo the health value of any salad by really ramping up the calories. Because it's drenched with dressing, Caesar salad is usually loaded with fat and calories. If you must have it, order dressing on the side and use sparingly. A Greek salad that's overflowing with feta cheese and olives will also be loaded with fat and calories. Ask for half the cheese, limit yourself to a few olives, and use a low-fat dressing.

Pizza. Avoid "deep dish," "stuffed crust," "extra cheese," and all other manner of hyperfattening pizza (including pepperoni and sausage, which should be limited to the occasional splurge). The calories are usually beyond comprehension. If you must order it, eat it plain (cheese only) or with vegetable toppings like spinach, mushrooms, broccoli, and roasted peppers. Portion control is key. It will be easier to limit yourself to a slice or two if you also order a large salad with low-fat dressing to help fill you up.

Pasta. Choose tomato-based marinara or primavera sauces rather than cream-based sauces. Tomato sauce delivers a fraction of the calories of cream sauce and actually counts as a vegetable serving! Be brave and ask for half the plate to be covered with the vegetable of the day. Halving your plate of pasta will halve your carbs for the meal. Try covering the veggies with tomato sauce to trick your brain into thinking you've had a full plate of pasta.

Soups. Broth-based soups are low in calories and make a great premeal filler or can be part of a calorie-controlled entrée when paired with a salad. Creamed soups, bisques, and chowders are much higher in calories. Limit them to special occasions.

Seafood. Fish and seafood dishes are great for you if you order them baked, broiled, poached, steamed, grilled, or lightly sautéed. Although it is delicious, deep-frying seafood adds unhealthy saturated fats and can more than double the calories. Try to resist the side order of fries (remember: sweet potato fries are still fried). Instead, ask for an extra vegetable.

Vegetarian entrées. These can be great choices if they're not loaded with butter, cheese, and fried vegetables. They're more likely to include whole grains, beans, and other high-fiber foods. Be adventurous and try tofu. It takes on the flavor of whatever it's cooked in, so you might be pleasantly surprised! Remain mindful of portions.

Burgers. Order the smallest burger on the menu (or try a turkey or veggie burger), watch the cheese and mayo, eat only half the bun, and ask for a salad to replace the giant side of fries. A typical fast-food hamburger (about the size of what you'd find in a child's meal) is about 300 calories, 10 to 15 grams of fat, and 35 grams of carbohydrate. From there, the sky's the limit as to what else might be loaded on the burger.

Mexican food. Ask your server not to bring fried tortilla chips to the table. Look for whole wheat tortillas, beans, and grilled entrées on the menu. Steer clear of deep-fried entrées like chimichangas and dishes with tons of cheese and sour cream. If you order a taco salad, don't eat the fried shell.

Speak Up and Ask the Staff

Don't be shy about talking to the wait staff, restaurant manager, or chef for advice on which menu items best meet your needs and preferences. If you don't know how something is prepared, ask. Request that your entrée be prepared with less fat or salt. Make substitutions to lower the carb or calorie content of the meal. Restaurants are part of the hospitality industry—they want you to come back, so most will go above and beyond to please.

Other helpful hints: Limit yourself to one piece of bread or skip it altogether. Avoid fatty breads like croissants, sweet rolls, and gooey pastries. Experiment with ethnic fare, which often uses unique spices and fresh herb blends to season foods, relying less on salt and fat. The same principles apply, however: if you don't know what's in it, ask. Always be on the lookout for fried and other high-fat foods, curb your carb intake, and search the menu for extra vegetables.

Dessert. Try your best to look beyond the chocolate cake and ice cream sundaes—the amount of carbohydrate they add to your meal can send your insulin levels sky-high. If you decide to go for it, ask someone to split the treat with you or—even better—suggest a dessert that the whole table can share.

Beverages. Beverages can add an insane number of calories to a meal if you're not careful. Choose water, diet soda, seltzer water with lemon or lime, low-fat milk, tea, or coffee in place of soda or other sweetened drinks. If consumed at all, limit alcohol-containing drinks to one per day for women, two for men.

Part 5

PREVENTING DIABETES WITH A HEALTHY MIND-SET

14

Managing Emotions
for Success

Without question, being diagnosed with prediabetes is stressful, and some research has tried to tie psychological stress to increased risk of diabetes. A complicating factor is that those who lead stressful lives often have difficulty practicing positive health behaviors, which in turn raises risk. Rather than adding fear of stress worsening your prediabetes to your list of things to worry about, work on replacing the negative feelings about all the things you should be doing but aren't with steps you can take to feel more in control of your schedule, habits, and health.

Changing lifestyle behaviors is extremely challenging: it requires deconstructing unhealthy habits and replacing them with healthier ones that stick. But the changes don't need to happen all at once. In the insightful words of my professional mentor, Dr. Margo Woods, a nutrition professor and researcher at the world-renowned Tufts University School of Nutrition in Boston: "Research shows dietary change is a three-step process that people need to move through, but often quit when they're only halfway there!" As we explored in part 1 of this book, those steps look roughly like this: Step one is to cut out the junk food. Step two is to start experimenting with healthier foods. Step three is to practice the new habits consistently.

To avoid feeling overwhelmed, start with one food and one exercise goal. Pick things that are realistic so you start racking up positive achievements that will empower you to continue. Maybe start by cooking a large meal on Sunday so you have healthy leftovers for a couple of nights this week. Or set a goal to walk twenty minutes—just open the door, walk out ten minutes, then turn around and walk back. Tell yourself you can do this. It's okay to work toward goals in your own way and at your own pace. Replace the old voices in your head that may be telling you that you *can't* with new positive messages that you *can*. If making changes in the food realm paralyzes you, start with increasing your activity. Exercise helps ease stress, anxiety, and depression in a number of incredibly powerful ways. It does all of the following:

- Increases production of feel-good neurotransmitters and endorphins (responsible for that "runner's high" people talk about).
- Blunts the release of immune system chemicals that can aggravate depression.
- Increases body temperature, which can have a calming effect.
- Provides a socially appropriate means of working off negative energy.
- Removes chemical by-products of the body's fight-or-flight stress response by simulating the activity that is fed by this reaction, thereby helping the body recover faster from this instinctive stress response.
- Helps increase self-confidence in what you think your body is capable of—strength and cardio fitness feel terrific!
- Gets you in touch with your muscles from the neck down, many of which may not have been used in years. This may improve self-esteem and how you feel about your appearance.
- Distracts you from what's troubling you, potentially short-circuiting a cycle of negative thoughts.
- Provides structure to your day, which may help you stay on track with eating as well.
- May improve your self-confidence so that you can tackle the challenges of healthy eating as well!

People who feel stressed or depressed may also feel socially isolated, and exercise gets you out in the world. Group exercise offers many benefits beyond physical. If you go to a gym or exercise class at the same time often enough, you may start to connect with others who have similar goals. Even better for accountability is finding a supportive exercise buddy. Also, for many people, *not* exercising is a source of stress because you know you should but aren't. Getting up and moving can relieve the anxiety that you're not taking care of yourself.

De-Stressing Indulgences

Beyond establishing a regular exercise routine, take advantage of other therapies available in today's wellness industry. Massage therapy, qigong, acupuncture, Reiki, aromatherapy, meditation, prayer, art, music, and dance can help you feel relaxed and give you a chance to appreciate what it means to feel good. This is what we mean by the "mind-body connection." Include some of these indulgences in your physical and emotional health improvement plan.

Developing an "I Can Change" Mind-Set

When it comes to changing routine behaviors, slow and steady really does win the race. Behavior change is a process, not an event. Rather than picking a day to jump in and try to change everything at once, in the long term it's more effective—and less stressful—to take on a new behavior or two and practice them for a while until they become familiar and more routine. You can then take on another healthy habit, working down your list of behaviors you'd like to change over time. If you're persistent enough, these new routines will eventually become just the way you do things.

For many people, the first step in changing behavior is to work on halting negative self-talk. People really are capable of change. In the case of weight loss, you can see this in the findings of the National Weight Control Registry, a database of more than ten thousand people who have lost an average of sixty-six pounds and kept it off for an average of 5.5 years. Remember the wise words of Dr. Margo Woods: "Dietary change is a three-step process that people need to move through." Let's take a look at these three steps in greater detail.

Step 1. Purge the refined foods from your diet (and kitchen cabinets!). These are foods that are filling you up and racking up the calories but aren't making any positive nutritional contributions to your diet. These foods include sweets, sugary beverages, salty snacks, fatty or fried foods, fast foods, and white-flour refined carbs. It's not that you have to avoid these foods altogether; they just need to be moved to your "eat less often" or "special occasions" list, and not making them too easily available is a good first start.

Step 2. Start overhauling the nutritional quality of one meal or snack at a time. Substitute a nonfat Greek yogurt or some hummus and carrots

Mind-Set Intervention: Change Is Always Emotional

Changing your eating and exercise habits is not just about knowing what you need to do. It's about learning new habits and strategies that help you evolve to a healthier place. No matter how smart or accomplished you are in other aspects of your life, this can be hard. Making diet and lifestyle changes is largely an emotional process. It's important to shake off your past experiences and expectations of weight loss and accept that it comes from making permanent change—not from temporarily following an overrestrictive diet plan.

One obstacle to successful weight loss is unrealistic expectations about how fast you should expect to lose weight, particularly if you lost a lot of weight quickly during a past weight-loss attempt. Immersing yourself in the latest popular diet program with the hope that if you just stick to the rules, no matter how restrictive, they will eventually become second nature, is a failing plan. The weight you might have lost using those methods was just sitting on the sidelines, waiting for you to drift back to the lifestyle habits that didn't serve you well before the diet.

Slower weight loss may be more likely to be permanent because it tends to reflect that you're making gradual, cumulative changes. You are transitioning from an old set of unhealthy habits to some healthier new ones. But you don't have to be perfect! I'm a big believer in the 80/20 rule: I care about what my patients do 80 percent of the time, as that tends to reflect their routines and habits. It also leaves room for some special treats and the occasional "out-of-the-ordinary" food experience. Success comes from repetition and being willing to try again even when all you seem to notice are your mistakes.

for that afternoon vending-machine snack. Replace that candy bar with a fruit salad. Switch out the full-fat salad dressing from the office cafeteria with some reduced-fat dressing that you bring from home. If you keep at these one-at-a-time changes, the overall quality of your diet will start to look different, and you will eventually arrive at step 3.

Step 3. Start to eat a consistently healthier diet. For the prediabetes diet plan, this means three meals a day plus one or two snacks (as needed to manage hunger) of whole, unrefined foods—whole grain breads, cereals, and crackers; whole fruits; lots of vegetables; low- or reduced-fat dairy; and reasonably sized portions (generally 3 to 6 ounces) of seafood, poultry, or lean meat, maybe including a vegetarian meal once or twice a week. It's still okay to incorporate a small portion of something sweet (or some other special treat) here and there. You just need to keep a realistic eye on how many calories these treats are contributing to your diet, and how many healthier foods they may be nudging out.

Unfortunately, in today's quick-fix society, many people start to lose their focus at step 2. We're impatient because we aren't losing enough weight or seeing a fast enough improvement in our blood sugars, or we're simply not used to this gradual approach.

But hitting step 3 is where the rewards start kicking in—where you actually start to look and feel differently in your body. There will be struggles and lapses, but hang in there! Without a doubt, eating healthier in our junk food–infused culture requires getting used to a little discomfort because it requires restraint. But if you've tried to change your diet and lifestyle habits many times before without lasting success and now your health is at stake, do you really have a choice? What is there to lose by spending the next few months trying to settle in with some new habits instead of steadily increasing your blood sugar, gaining more weight, or feeling progressively uncomfortable—and unhappy?

Rally the Troops: Know When to Ask for Help

If your readiness to take charge of your prediabetes is there, identify the supports you need and don't be afraid to ask for help. I once read somewhere that stress is not an outside force you find threatening, but your response to it. Finding a way to change how you respond to stress is an important part of feeling more in control of your life. By all means, seek out support—from a registered dietitian, a doctor, a certified diabetes educator, a weight-loss support group, or an online chat room. Support is vital for helping you get back in the saddle when you fall off and are tempted to stay lying in the dirt. Don't be afraid to admit you might need psychological therapy to deal with your food or "resistance-to-change" issues. These are common and therapy can be life changing. Many of our most self-destructive thought processes have been reinforced for years, and we may benefit from the help of a professional to untangle and rewire these messages.

15

Devising Your Own Prediabetes Diet Plan

Managing and perhaps reversing your prediabetes through diet and lifestyle change is absolutely possible. *The Prediabetes Diet Plan* has clarified what prediabetes is, how it affects your health, and how it can be treated to reduce your risk of developing full-blown diabetes. Most important, receiving a diagnosis of prediabetes presents an opportunity to finally work on changing habits and routines that are threatening your health and quality of life. This book makes the case for *why* what you do with food, activity, and lifestyle choices makes a difference. Remember:

- The food choices you make can either aggravate your insulin resistance or improve it.
- Physical activity is "natural medicine" for insulin resistance and is essential for weight loss and stress management.
- Sensible dietary supplementation can optimize the nutrient profile of your diet for better health, but supplementation is not a substitute for healthy eating.
- Tending to your emotional needs is essential to overall health and can make picking a plan and sticking with it more achievable.

Much of what people read about diet and nutrition is confusing. They want to eat better but don't really know how to do it—and this can become yet one more obstacle. Following the prediabetes diet plan makes it easier to implement healthy changes. Another obstacle is the commonly held belief that eating well is an all-or-nothing prospect: if you can't change radically all at once (the traditional approach to weight loss), why bother changing at all? But research shows this is not how people change their

Mind-Set Intervention: It's Okay to Start Small

Counting carbs, considering exchange lists, tightening up portions—there is a lot to take in once you've committed to managing your prediabetes through a healthy diet. But that's why you have options. In the beginning you might just start eating off a smaller plate, aiming for the balanced-plate approach without counting carbs. Just trading off that extra portion of rice for a serving of vegetables and throwing the rest of your energy at increasing your activity may be as far as you go in the first few weeks. If you find you need some help with carb portions, however, carb counting is likely to be beneficial. But you don't need to jump right in. Test the waters by paying some extra attention to your eating pattern. Make an effort to eat your next meal or snack before you're starving. Then start adding more vegetables to your dinner plate. Lasting behavior change comes from trekking your own path at your own pace. Even with slow progress, within a year's time you'll likely be slimmer and healthier—and less likely to have progressed toward diabetes than you are today.

habits long term. Slow and steady change suggests you're doing the hard work of looking at your diet and lifestyle habits one at a time and experimenting with ways you can change them permanently.

Being realistic about how long it will take to change those habits is important. You didn't develop your current habits overnight, and it will take time to establish new ones. Crash diets make false promises about overnight, painless transformation, but anyone who has tried one of those methods can tell you that they rarely work long term. Eventually you get sick of the shakes or bars or overly restrictive meal plans and end up in a place where you have two choices: (1) do nothing and continue on a path of discontent and concern about your health, or (2) start chipping away at it in a positive direction. Your path may be tediously slow, addressing one habit, meal, or task at a time. Or maybe you've decided, "This is it, I'm ready," and you move along at a steady, determined pace. However you choose to go about it, you may find it helpful to recall the ten strategies for weight loss and lifestyle change outlined in detail in chapter 8 and listed again here in brief.

Strategy #1: Learn how your body works. Being strongly attracted to food and squirreling away excess calories is natural for our primitive genetic design, making it easy to overeat and gain weight. Work with your genes rather than against them by prioritizing eating before you're starved, and cover half your plate with whole fruits and vegetables that will fill you up without loading you down with excess calories.

Strategy #2: Adjust your attitude. One of the hardest things to do is believe that you are capable of making change. Historically, diets have been about being either 100 percent "in" or "out" without room for lapses along the way. Accept that this isn't realistic, and know that lapses are opportunities to learn, not evidence of weakness or failure.

Strategy #3: Keep a food journal. Keeping a journal—whether pen-to-paper or an online website or app—is one of the most helpful things you can do to keep track of what's really happening with your food choices and enhance your accountability. Don't think of it as something that's not worth doing if you can't commit to it every day. Do what you can and see what happens.

Strategy #4: Avoid overeating at night. Recent research supports what many nutritionists have known for a long time—eating too much at night may make it easier to gain weight. At a minimum, start out with a healthy breakfast and avoid eating too little during the busy part of the day. It's a classic setup for hunger—and portions—to spin out of control from mid- to late afternoon on.

Strategy #5: Budget time for self-care. Diet and lifestyle change takes time and energy, as well as some swimming upstream against societal norms. Try to accept that despite the sacrifices in the end it will be worth it. Making changes that lead to a better quality of life is an incredible gift to give yourself and your family.

Strategy #6: Manage your hunger to control portions. Relying on will-power and good intentions to help you avoid overeating when you're over-hungry is likely to fail. Work toward being a proactive eater by eating your next meal or snack before you're starved. It may help you make healthier choices and slow you down a little.

Strategy #7: Make losing weight a priority. We can always find "screen-time" to watch TV or search the Internet. Work toward budgeting in some "me time" to tend to your personal health needs, like food shopping, cooking, and exercise.

Strategy #8: Manage your expectations. It can be incredibly tough to avoid lapsing into our usual thinking patterns about weight loss and diet change. Hopefully the different angle presented by *The Prediabetes Diet*

Plan—which encourages a positive approach to managing insulin resistance instead of "dieting"—will provide a unique perspective that helps you avoid the usual emotional potholes and unrealistic expectations.

Strategy #9: Don't go it alone. No one is an island. Seek out support—from a family member, friend, coworker, counselor, or group. It's been proven to enhance success, and makes the road to change seem less lonely and more fun!

Strategy #10: Be patient. We're an impatient population, and with diet and behavior change we're no different. Try to accept that it probably took years to get where you are, and that tossing out unhealthful habits and replacing them with better ones takes time.

Perfection Is the Enemy of "Good Enough"

Clearly, change isn't easy, and there are challenges along the way. Some may relate to your living situation—maybe you're ready to start eating healthier, but your partner isn't. Or after working a long day, possibly topped off with a long commute, it's hard for you to prioritize meal planning or exercise. For many of us, the obstacles are emotional. You may have a decades-old habit of overeating in response to stress or disappointment, or feel like you've failed at trying to lose weight and eat more healthfully so many times that you're terrified to try again. Or maybe you're just not ready. But remember the old adage that "perfection is the enemy of good enough." Just because you don't have readiness to make major moves to live a healthier life doesn't mean setting a goal or two isn't worth it. I hope reading this book will move you a little closer to readiness—and that is progress.

There will always be uncertainties in managing prediabetes, but making any move, no matter how small, toward leading a healthier life will empower you to feel like you're not just waiting for doctors to make you feel better. You're pitching it, taking charge, and hedging your bets that trying something new is better than doing nothing at all. Everyone's journey with prediabetes is unique and there are many paths. Your journey will happen at the pace that is right for you. It is my hope that the prediabetes diet plan will help you see that small changes over time can make a big difference to your health and quality of life. Why not start today?

Appendix 1: Sample Meal Plans

The meal plans provided here are designed to provide a framework for a new way of eating, and help you develop a sense of how much carbohydrate you should try to limit yourself to per meal based on your estimated calorie needs. There are three days of meal plans for four different calorie levels: 1500, 1700, 2000, and 2300 calories. Because we use the American Diabetes Association's Exchange Lists as the foundation for our discussion on carbohydrate counting, for the nutrient analysis these meal plans list the "grams of carbohydrate" exactly as they appear in the American Diabetes Association Exchange Lists for Diabetes. This includes counting the carbohydrates in non-starchy vegetables, and considers a serving of milk or unsweetened yogurt to contain 12 grams of carbohydrate, whereas for our purposes we round the carbohydrate content to 15 grams to keep things simple. In our prediabetes diet plan we are using the Exchange Lists as a tool to help people who are not diabetic develop a sense of carbohydrate servings, which allows us some flexibility in utilizing the lists (so we consider carbs from nonstarchy vegetables "free" and round milk and yogurt carbs to 15 grams per serving). If you are diabetic, you should seek out the advice of a registered dietitian to determine how to best manage your carbohydrate intake to control your blood glucose and work with your medications.

To clarify what we are "counting" for the prediabetes diet plan, the far right column lists the number of carb choices, which includes carb choices from starches (including starchy vegetables), fruit, milk/yogurt and sweets (though we are allowing up to a teaspoon of added sugar to be "free"), and excludes nonstarchy vegetables. Under the grams of carbohydrate column, each meal lists the carbs for each food in the meal, and then the total carbs for each meal, using the Exchange Lists carbohydrate numbers. Because in this column we are counting all the carbs as presented in the Exchange Lists you will notice these numbers do not add up to exactly between 45 and 75 grams, but they're in the range (sometimes a little higher or lower). This is fine as we're looking to estimate the amount of carbohydrate eaten per meal without becoming overwhelmed with the details.

To make these plans work for you, if you note a food choice that isn't your preference (for example, a vegetable or protein choice you don't eat), simply refer to the exchange lists and replace it with a food you like. Even though proteins and fats don't contain carbohydrates (unless they're part of a combination food that does), it's still important to watch your portions if you're also trying to control your calorie intake.

1500-CALORIE MENUS   DAY ONE

MEAL	FOOD ITEM	SERVING SIZE	GRAMS OF CARBOHYDRATE
Breakfast			
	Old-fashioned oats (cook in water)	1 cup	30
	Brown sugar*	1 teaspoon	5
	Raisins	2 tablespoons	15
	Skim milk	8 fluid ounces	12
			62 g Carb
Morning snack			
	Apple	1, small	15
			15 g Carb
Lunch			
	Salad greens	2 cups	10
	Sliced tomatoes	½ cup	2.5
	Sliced carrots	½ cup	2.5
	Feta cheese	1 ounce	0
	Grilled chicken breast (skinless)	3 ounces	0
	Sunflower seeds	2 tablespoons	4
	Salad dressing	2 tablespoons	0
	Walnuts, shelled & halved	12 halves	4
	Whole grain dinner roll	1, small	15
			38 g Carb
Afternoon snack			
	Nonfat Greek yogurt (vanilla)	6 ounces	13
	Raspberries	1 cup	15
			28 g Carb
Dinner			
	Whole wheat pasta (cooked)	1 cup	30
	Tomato sauce	1 cup	10
	Meatball	1 ounce	0
	Parmesan cheese	2 teaspoons	0
	Cauliflower	1 cup	10
			50 g Carb
		TOTALS	**198 g Carb**
			49%

* This small amount of sugar is counted as free.

GRAMS OF PROTEIN	GRAMS OF FAT	GRAMS OF FIBER	TOTAL CALORIES	# OF CARB "CHOICES"
5	3	5	150	2
0	0	0	16	-
0	0	1	60	1
8	0	0	90	1
13 g Protein	**3 g Fat**	**6 g Fiber**	**316 Calories**	**4**
0	0	3	60	1
		3 g Fiber	**60 Calories**	**1**
4	0	5	50	-
1	0	1	12	-
1	0	1	12	-
7	5	0	75	-
21	3	0	105	-
3	8	1	90	-
0	10	0	90	-
4	16	2	160	-
3	0	2	80	1
44 g Protein	**42 g Fat**	**12 g Fiber**	**674 Calories**	**1**
16	0	0	120	1
0	0	3	60	1
16 g Protein		**3 g Fiber**	**180 Calories**	**2**
6	1	4	160	2
4	0	4	50	-
7	5	0	75	-
1	2	0	20	-
4	0	5	50	-
22 g Protein	**8 g Fat**	**13 g Fiber**	**355 Calories**	**2**
95 g Protein	**53 g Fat**	**37 g Fiber**	**1585 Calories**	**10**
24%	**30%**			

MEAL	FOOD ITEM	SERVING SIZE	GRAMS OF CARBOHYDRA
Breakfast			
	Shredded wheat cereal	1 cup (2 biscuits)	30
	Skim mlk	8 fluid ounces	12
	Blueberries, fresh or frozen	¾ cup	15
	Almonds, unsalted, roasted	6 almonds	0
			57 g Carb
Morning snack			
	Orange	1, small	15 g
			15 g Carb
Lunch			
	100% whole wheat bread	2 slices	30
	Turkey breast, sliced	2 ounces	0
	American cheese	1-ounce slice	0
	Roasted red pepper hummus	2 tablespoons	3
	Sliced tomato	3, ½-inch thick	3
	Salad greens	¼ cup	2.5
	Apple	1, small	15
			54 g Carb
Afternoon snack			
	String cheese	1-ounce stick	0
	Whole wheat crackers	5	15
			15 g Carb
Dinner			
	Pork tenderloin (garlic & herb)	3 ounces	0
	Olive oil	1 tablespoon	0
	Baked potato	1, med. (5 ounces)	30
	Butter/margarine spread	1 teaspoon	0
	Broccoli, steamed	1 cup	10
			40 g Carb
		TOTALS	**181 g Carb**
			48%

GRAMS OF PROTEIN	GRAMS OF FAT	GRAMS OF FIBER	TOTAL CALORIES	# OF CARB "CHOICES"
5	1	6	160	2
8	0	0	90	1
0	0	3	60	1
2	5	1	45	-
15 g Protein	**6 g Fat**	**10 g Fiber**	**355 Calories**	**4**
0	0	3	60	1
		3 g Fiber	**60 Calories**	**1**
8	2	4	100	2
14	2	0	70	-
7	8	0	100	-
1	6	1	70	-
0	0	1	15	-
1	0	1	12	-
0	0	3	60	1
31 g Protein	**18 g Fat**	**10 g Fiber**	**427 Calories**	**3**
8	5	0	80	-
3	0	2	80	1
11 g Protein	**5 g Fat**	**2 g Fiber**	**160 Calories**	**1**
21	9	0	165	-
0	14	0	120	-
3	0	3	130	2
0	5	0	45	-
4	0	6	50	-
28 g Protein	**28 g Fat**	**9 g Fiber**	**510 Calories**	**2**
85 g Protein	**57 g Fat**	**34 g Fiber**	**1512 Calories**	**11**
22%	**34%**			

MEAL	FOOD ITEM	SERVING SIZE	GRAMS OF CARBOHYDRA
Breakfast			
	100% whole wheat toast	1 slice	15
	Butter/margarine spread	1 teaspoon	0
	Eggs, cooked without fat	2 large	0
	Nonfat greek yogurt	6 ounces	12
	Strawberries, whole, fresh	1¼ cups	15
			42 g Carb
Morning snack			
	Grapes	17 grapes	15
			15 g Carb
Lunch			
	Thin-crust cheese pizza	¼ of 12-inch pie	30
	Toppings: (measured raw)		5
	Sliced orange bell pepper	¼ cup	
	Sliced red onion	¼ cup	
	Spinach	¼ cup	
	Sliced red bell pepper	¼ cup	
	Mini tangerines (fresh)	2	15
			50 g Carb
Afternoon snack			
	Carrot sticks	1 cup	5
	Hummus	¼ cup	8
			13 g Carb
Dinner			
	Lentil soup	1½ cups	45
	Whole grain dinner roll	1, small	15
	Parmesan cheese	4 teaspoons	0
			60 g Carb
		TOTALS	**180 g Carb**
			51%

GRAMS OF PROTEIN	GRAMS OF FAT	GRAMS OF FIBER	TOTAL CALORIES	# OF CARB "CHOICES"
4	1	2	50	1
0	5	0	45	-
14	10	0	150	-
16	0	0	120	1
0	0	3	60	1
34 g Protein	**16 g Fat**	**5 g Fiber**	**425 Calories**	**3**
0	0	2	60	1
		2 g Fiber	**60 Calories**	**1**
20	15	0	355	2
2	0	3	25	-
				-
				-
				-
				-
0	0	2	60	1
22 g Protein	**15 g Fat**	**5 g Fiber**	**440 Calories**	**3**
2	0	2	25	0
4	6	4	90	⅔
6 g Protein	**6 g Fat**	**6 g Fiber**	**115 Calories**	**1**
13.5	3	7.5	240	2
3	0	2	80	1
2	4	0	40	-
18.5 g Protein	**7 g Fat**	**9.5 g Fiber**	**360 Calories**	**3**
80.5 g Protein	**44 g Fat**	**27.5 g Fiber**	**1400 Calories**	**11**
23%	**28%**			

1700-CALORIE MENUS   **DAY ONE**

MEAL	FOOD ITEM	SERVING SIZE	GRAMS OF CARBOHYDRATE
Breakfast			
	100% whole wheat toast	2 slices	30
	Butter/margarine spread	1 teaspoon	0
	Egg, cooked without fat	2 large	0
	1% milk	8 fluid ounces	12
	Cantaloupe, cubed	1 cup	15
			57 g Carb
Morning snack			
	Raspberries, fresh or frozen	1 cup	15
			15 g Carb
Lunch			
	Chicken noodle soup (low sodium)	1 cup	15
	Salad greens	2 cups	10
	Sliced tomatoes	½ cup	2.5
	Sliced carrots	½ cup	2.5
	Salad dressing	2 tablespoons	0
	100% whole wheat bread	1 slice	15
	Cheddar cheese (or other similar type)	1 ounce	0
			45 g Carb
Afternoon snack			
	Nonfat greek yogurt (plain)	6 ounces	12
	Blueberries (fresh or frozen)	¾ cup	15
			27 g Carb
Dinner			
	Baked potato	1, med. (5 ounces)	30
	Cheddar cheese (shredded)	1 ounce	0
	Grilled chicken (with herbs)	3 ounces	0
	Steamed carrots	1 cup	10
	Green grapes	17 grapes	15
			55 g Carb
		TOTALS	**199 g Carb**
			48%

GRAMS OF PROTEIN	GRAMS OF FAT	GRAMS OF FIBER	TOTAL CALORIES	# OF CARB "CHOICES"
8	2	4	100	2
0	5	0	45	-
14	10	0	150	-
8	2.5	0	130	1
0	0	2	60	1
30 g Protein	**19.5 g Fat**	**6 g Fiber**	**485 Calories**	**4**
0	0	2	60	1
		2 g Fiber	**60 Calories**	**1**
6	2	1	90	1
4	0	5	50	-
1	0	1	12	-
1	0	1	12	-
0	10	0	90	-
4	1	2	50	1
7	8	0	100	-
23 g Protein	**21 g Fat**	**10 g Fiber**	**404 Calories**	**2**
16	0	0	120	1
0	0	3	60	1
16 g Protein		**2 g Fiber**	**180 Calories**	**2**
3	0	3	130	2
7	8	0	100	-
21	9	0	165	-
4	0	6	50	-
0	0	2	60	1
35 g Protein	**17 g Fat**	**11 g Fiber**	**505 Calories**	**3**
104 g Protein	**57.5 g Fat**	**31 g Fiber**	**1634 Calories**	**12**
25%	**32%**			

DAY TWO

1700-CALORIE MENUS

MEAL	FOOD ITEM	SERVING SIZE	GRAMS OF CARBOHYDRATE
Breakfast			
	Old-fashioned oats (cook in water)	1 cup	30
	Banana, mashed in oatmeal	1 small	15
	Walnuts, shelled & halved	12 halves	4
	Skim milk	8 fluid ounces	12
			61 g Carb
Morning snack			
	Pineapple, cubed	¾ cup	15
			15 g Carb
Lunch			
	Pita bread pocket, whole wheat	6-inch piece	30
	Hummus	2 tablespoons	4
	Roasted turkey breast	2 ounces	0
	Lettuce	½ cup	3
	Sliced tomato	3, ½-inch thick	3
	Apple	1, small	15
			55 g Carb
Afternoon snack			
	Low-fat Cheddar cheese	2 ounces	0
	Whole wheat crackers	5	15
			15 g Carb
Dinner			
	Salmon	4 ounces	0
	Olive oil	2 teaspoons	0
	Roasted carrots	½ cup	5
	Steamed broccoli	½ cup	5
	Cheddar cheese	1 ounce	0
	Brown rice	⅔ cup	30
			40 g Carb
		TOTALS	**186 g Carb**
			45%

GRAMS OF PROTEIN	GRAMS OF FAT	GRAMS OF FIBER	TOTAL CALORIES	# OF CARB "CHOICES"
5	3	5	150	2
0	0	3	60	1
4	16	2	160	-
8	0	0	90	1
17 g Protein	**19 g Fat**	**10 g Fiber**	**460 Calories**	**4**
0	0	2	60	1
		2 g Fiber	**60 Calories**	**1**
6	2	5	170	2
2	3	2	45	-
14	1	0	75	-
1	0	2	13	-
0	0	1	15	-
0	0	2	60	1
23 g Protein	**6 g Fat**	**12 g Fiber**	**378 Calories**	**3**
14	4	0	100	-
3	0	2	80	1
17 g Protein	**4 g Fat**	**2 g Fiber**	**180 Calories**	**1**
28	12	0	220	-
0	7	0	60	-
2	0	3	25	-
2	0	3	25	-
7	8	0	100	-
6	0	4	160	2
45 g Protein	**27 g Fat**	**10 g Fiber**	**590 Calories**	**2**
102 g Protein	**56 g Fat**	**36 g Fiber**	**1668 Calories**	**11**
24%	**30%**			

DAY THREE

1700-CALORIE MENUS

MEAL	FOOD ITEM	SERVING SIZE	GRAMS OF CARBOHYDRATE
Breakfast			
	Bran flakes	1 cup	30
	Raisins	2 tablespoons	15
	1% milk	8 fluid ounces	12
	Almonds, unsalted, roasted	12 almonds	0
			57 g Carb
Morning snack			
	Strawberries, whole, fresh	1¼ cups	15
			15 g Carb
Lunch			
	100% whole wheat bread	2 slices	30
	Tuna, canned in water	3 ounces	0
	Olive oil mayonnaise	2 tablespoons	1
	Lettuce	½ cup	3
	Sliced tomato	3, ½-inch thick	3
	Apple	1, small	15
			51 g Carb
Afternoon snack			
	Nonfat greek yogurt (fruit flavored)	6 ounces	20
			20 g Carb
Dinner			
	Turkey & bean chili	1 cup	25
	Brown rice	⅔ cup	30
	Pepper Jack cheese	2 ounces	0
	Salad greens	1 cup	5
	Sliced tomatoes	½ cup	2.5
	Sliced carrots	½ cup	2.5
	Salad dressing	2 tablespoons	0
			65 g Carb
		TOTALS	**208 g Carb**
			47%

GRAMS OF PROTEIN	GRAMS OF FAT	GRAMS OF FIBER	TOTAL CALORIES	# OF CARB "CHOICES"
4	1	7	160	2
0	0	1	60	1
8	2.5	0	130	1
4	10	2	90	-
16 g Protein	**13.5 g Fat**	**10 g Fiber**	**440 Calories**	**4**
0	0	3	60	1
0 g Protein	**0 g Fat**	**3 g Fiber**	**60 Calories**	**1**
8	2	4	100	2
21	2	0	105	-
0	10	0	100	-
1	0	2	13	-
0	0	1	15	-
0	0	3	60	1
30 g Protein	**19 g Fat**	**10 g Fiber**	**428 Calories**	**3**
14	0	0	140	1
14 g Protein			**140 Calories**	**about 1**
16	3	6	193	2
6	0	4	160	2
10	16	0	216	-
2	0	2	25	-
1	0	1	12	-
1	0	1	12	-
0	10	0	90	-
36 g Protein	**29 g Fat**	**14 g Fiber**	**708 Calories**	**4**
96 g Protein	**61.5 g Fat**	**37 g Fiber**	**1776 Calories**	**13**
22%	**31%**			

MEAL	FOOD ITEM	SERVING SIZE	GRAMS OF CARBOHYDRA*
Breakfast			
	Whole wheat English muffin	1 whole	30
	Peanut butter	2 tablespoons	8
	Eggs, scrambled	2	0
	Banana	1, small	15
			53 g Carb
Morning snack			
	Cherries, fresh	24	30
			30 g Carb
Lunch			
	Grilled cheese sandwich:		
	100% whole wheat bread	2 slices	30
	American cheese (2% milk fat)	2 slices	4
	Salad greens	1 cup	5
	Sliced tomatoes	½ cup	2.5
	Sliced carrots	½ cup	2.5
	Beans, garbanzo	½ cup	21
	Salad dressing	2 tablespoons	0
			65 g Carb
Afternoon snack			
	Nonfat greek yogurt (fruit flavored)	6 ounces	20
			20 g Carb
Dinner			
	Baked Swordfish (lemon & herb seasoning)	4 ounces	0
	Bread crumbs	¼ cup	20
	Olive oil	2 teaspoons	0
	Baked sweet potato	1 medium	30
	Olive oil/butter spread	1 tablespoon	0
	Steamed asparagus	1 cup	10
			60 g Carb
Evening snack			
	Almonds, unsalted, roasted	6 almonds	0
	Grapes	17 grapes	15
			15 g Carb
		TOTALS	**243 g Carb**
			50%

GRAMS OF PROTEIN	GRAMS OF FAT	GRAMS OF FIBER	TOTAL CALORIES	# OF CARB "CHOICES"
5	1	3	130	2
7	16	2	190	-
14	10	0	150	-
0	0	3	60	1
26 g Protein	**27 g Fat**	**8 g Fiber**	**530 Calories**	**3**
0	0	5	120	2
		5 g Fiber	**120 Calories**	**2**
8	2	4	100	2
8	5	0	100	-
2	0	2	25	-
1	0	1	12.5	-
1	0	1	12.5	-
8	1	8	115	1
0	10	0	90	-
28 g Protein	**18 g Fat**	**16 g Fiber**	**455 Calories**	**3**
14	0	0	140	1
14 g Protein			**140 Calories**	**1**
30	6	0	175	-
3	1	1	100	about 1
0	7	0	60	-
2	0	4	120	2
0	7	0	60	-
4	0	3	50	-
39 g Protein	**21 g Fat**	**8 g Fiber**	**565 Calories**	**3**
2	5	1	45	-
0	0	2	60	1
2 g Protein	**5 g Fat**	**3 g Fiber**	**105 Calories**	**1**
109 g Protein	**71 g Fat**	**40 g Fiber**	**1915 Calories**	**13**
23%	**33%**			

MEAL	FOOD ITEM	SERVING SIZE	GRAMS OF CARBOHYDRAT
Breakfast			
	Whole wheat waffles	2	30
	Peanut butter	2 tablespoons	8
	Banana, sliced, top of waffles	1, small	15
	1% milk	8 fluid ounces	12
			65 g Carb
Morning snack			
	Raspberries	1 cup	15
	Blueberries	¾ cup	15
			30 g Carb
Lunch			
	Shrimp	3 ounces	0
	Stir-fried vegetables	1 cup cooked	10
	Olive oil	2 teaspoons	0
	Teriyaki sauce (reduced sodium)	2 tablespoons	6
	Brown rice	⅔ cup	30
	Orange	1, small	15
			61 g Carb
Afternoon snack			
	Whole wheat crackers	5	15
	Cheddar cheese	1 ounce	0
			15 g Carb
Dinner			
	Whole wheat pasta (cooked)	1 cup	45
	Tomato sauce (no sugar added)	½ cup	5
	Meatballs	3 (one ounce each)	0
	Parmesan cheese	2 teaspoons	0
	Steamed broccoli	1 cup	10
			60 g Carb
Evening snack			
	Plums	2, small	15
	Mixed nuts, roasted, no salt added	2 tablespoons	4
			19 g Carb
		TOTALS	**250 g Carb**
			49%

GRAMS OF PROTEIN	GRAMS OF FAT	GRAMS OF FIBER	TOTAL CALORIES	# OF CARB "CHOICES"
5	6	3	170	2
7	16	2	190	-
0	0	3	60	1
8	2.5	0	130	1
20 g Protein	**24.5 g Fat**	**8 g Fiber**	**550 Calories**	**4**
0	0	3	60	1
0	0	3	60	1
		6 g Fiber	**120 Calories**	**2**
21	2	0	105	-
4	0	3	50	-
0	7	0	60	-
0	1	0	30	-
6	0	5	160	2
0	0	2	60	1
31 g Protein	**10 g Fat**	**10 g Fiber**	**465 Calories**	**3**
3	0	2	80	1
7	9	0	115	-
10 g Protein	**9 g Fat**	**2 g Fiber**	**195 Calories**	**1**
8	1	4	200	3
4	0	4	25	-
21	15	0	225	-
1	2	0	20	-
4	0	3	50	-
36 g Protein	**18 g Fat**	**11 g Fiber**	**520 Calories**	**3**
0	0	4	60	1
3	10	2	110	-
3 g Protein	**10 g Fat**	**6 g Fiber**	**170 Calories**	**1**
100 g Protein	**71.5 g Fat**	**43 g Fiber**	**2020 Calories**	**14**
20%	**32%**			

MEAL	FOOD ITEM	SERVING SIZE	GRAMS OF CARBOHYDRATE
Breakfast			
	Shredded wheat cereal	1 cup (2 biscuits)	30
	1% milk	8 fluid ounces	12
	Blueberries, fresh or frozen	¾ cup	15
	Egg, hard-boiled	1, large	0
			57 g Carb
Morning snack			
	Apple	1, small	15
	Peanut butter	2 tablespoons	8
			23 g Carb
Lunch			
	Pita bread pocket, whole wheat	6-inch piece	30
	Hummus	2 tablespoons	4
	Roasted turkey breast	2 ounces	0
	Cheddar cheese	1 ounce	0
	Lettuce	½ cup	3
	Sliced tomato	3, ½-inch thick	3
	Apricot	1, small	15
			60 g Carb
Afternoon snack			
	Nonfat greek yogurt (plain)	6 ounces	13
	Blackberries	¾ cup	15
			28 g Carb
Dinner			
	Sirloin steak, grilled	4 ounces	0
	Baked potato	1, med. (5 ounces)	30
	Olive oil/butter spread	1 tablespoon	0
	Roasted brussels sprouts	1 cup, cooked	10
	Roasted carrots	1 cup, cooked	10
	Olive oil	2 teaspoons	0
			50 g Carb
Evening snack			
	Popcorn, air popped	3 cups	15
	Butter/margarine spread	2 teaspoons	0
	Sugar	1 teaspoon	4
	Cinnamon	dash	0
			19 g Carb
		TOTALS	**237 g Carb**
			47%

GRAMS OF PROTEIN	GRAMS OF FAT	GRAMS OF FIBER	TOTAL CALORIES	# OF CARB "CHOICES"
5	1	6	160	2
8	2.5	0	130	1
0	0	3	60	1
7	5	0	75	0
20 g Protein	**8.5 g Fat**	**9 g Fiber**	**425 Calories**	**4**
0	0	2	60	1
7	16	2	190	-
7 g Protein	**16 g Fat**	**4 g Fiber**	**60 Calories**	**1**
6	2	5	170	2
2	3	2	45	-
14	1	0	75	-
7	9	0	115	-
1	0	2	13	-
0	0	1	15	-
0	0	2	60	1
30 g Protein	**15 g Fat**	**12 g Fiber**	**493 Calories**	**3**
16	0	0	120	1
0	0	3	60	1
16 g Protein		**3 g Fiber**	**180 Calories**	**2**
21	9	0	165	-
3	0	3	130	2
0	7	0	60	-
4	0	3	55	-
4	0	3	55	-
0	7	0	60	-
32 g Protein	**23 g Fat**	**9 g Fiber**	**525 Calories**	**2**
2	0	2	45	1
0	10	0	90	-
0	0	0	16	-
0	0	0	0	-
2 g Protein	**5 g Fat**	**2 g Fiber**	**106 Calories**	**1**
107 g Protein	**72.5 g Fat**	**39 g Fiber**	**2024 Calories**	**13**
21%	**32%**			

MEAL	FOOD ITEM	SERVING SIZE	GRAMS OF CARBOHYDRA
Breakfast			
	Multigrain bagel	½ bagel	30
	Almond butter	1 tablespoon	3
	Strawberries, whole	1¼ cups	15
	Nonfat greek yogurt (plain)	6 ounces	13
	Eggs, hard boiled	2	0
			61 g Carb
Morning snack			
	Tangerines, small	2	15
			15 g Carb
Lunch			
	Whole wheat tortilla wrap	2 (6-inch) wraps	30
	Tuna, canned in water	5 ounces	0
	Mayonnaise	2 tablespoons	1
	Lettuce	½ cup	3
	Sliced tomato	3, ½-inch thick	3
	Avocado, sliced	⅓ cup	4
	Grapes	17 grapes	15
			56 g Carb
Afternoon snack			
	Low-fat cottage cheese, herb flavored	1 cup	6
	Multigrain crackers	10	30
			36 g Carb
Dinner			
	Pork tenderloin (roasted, seasoned with garlic, rosemary, thyme)	4 ounces	0
	Roasted pear	½ large	15
	Roasted potatoes	2, 3 ounces each	30
	Olive oil	1 tablespoon	0
	Steamed asparagus	1 cup	10
			55 g Carb
Evening snack			
	Blueberries (fresh or frozen)	¾ cup	15
	Granola	¼ cup	15
			30 g Carb
		TOTALS	**253 g Carb**
			44%

GRAMS OF PROTEIN	GRAMS OF FAT	GRAMS OF FIBER	TOTAL CALORIES	# OF CARB "CHOICES"
6	3	3	165	2
2	10	1	100	-
0	0	3	60	1
16	0	0	120	1
12	10	0	150	-
36 g Protein	**23 g Fat**	**7 g Fiber**	**595 Calories**	**4**
0	0	3	60	1
		3 g Fiber	**60 Calories**	**1**
4	2	3	160	2
35	3	0	175	-
0	10	0	100	-
1	0	2	13	-
0	0	1	15	-
1	7	3	80	-
0	0	2	60	1
41 g Protein	**22 g Fat**	**11 g Fiber**	**603 Calories**	**3**
28	2	0	160	-
6	0	4	160	2
34 g Protein	**2 g Fat**	**4 g Fiber**	**320 Calories**	**2**
28	12	0	220	-
0	0	3	60	1
6	0	3	160	2
0	14	0	120	-
4	0	3	50	-
38 g Protein	**26 g Fat**	**9 g Fiber**	**610 Calories**	**3**
0	0	3	60	1
3	5	2	125	1
3 g Protein	**5 g Fat**	**5 g Fiber**	**185 Calories**	**2**
152 g Protein	**78 g Fat**	**39 g Fiber**	**2373 Calories**	**15**
26%	**30%**			

MEAL	FOOD ITEM	SERVING SIZE	GRAMS OF CARBOHYDRAT
Breakfast			
	Bran flakes	1 cup	30
	Raisins	2 tablespoons	15
	1% milk	8 fluid ounces	12
	Canadian bacon	2 slices	0
	Egg, scrambled	1, large	0
			57 g Carb
Morning snack			
	Grapefruit	1, large	30
			30 g Carb
Lunch			
	Chicken noodle soup	1 cup	15
	Grilled cheese & tomato sandwich		
	100% whole wheat bread	2 slices	30
	Sliced tomato	3, ½-inch thick	3
	2% American cheese	2 slices	4
	Fruit salad	1 cup	30
			82 g Carb
Afternoon snack			
	100% whole wheat bread	1 slice	15
	Peanut butter	2 tablespoons	8
	Banana	1, small	15
			38 g Carb
Dinner			
	Ground turkey	4 ounces	0
	Taco seasoning, reduced sodium	1 tablespoon	5
	Corn tortilla	3 (6" across)	45
	Salsa	¼ cup	5
	Lettuce	½ cup	2.5
	Tomato, diced	½ cup	2.5
	Cheddar cheese (shredded)	1 ounce	0
	Refried beans	½ cup	15
			75 g Carb
Evening snack			
	Popcorn, air popped	3 cups	15
	Butter/margarine spread	2 teaspoons	0
			15 g Carb
		TOTALS	**297 g Carb**
			51%

GRAMS OF PROTEIN	GRAMS OF FAT	GRAMS OF FIBER	TOTAL CALORIES	# OF CARB "CHOICES"
4	1	7	160	2
0	0	1	60	1
8	2.5	0	130	1
12	4	0	90	-
6	5	0	75	-
30 g Protein	**12.5 g Fat**	**8 g Fiber**	**515 Calories**	**4**
0	0	3	120	2
		3 g Fiber	**120 Calories**	**2**
8	3	2	120	1
8	2	4	100	2
0	0	1	15	-
8	5	0	100	-
0	0	3	120	-
24 g Protein	**10 g Fat**	**10 g Fiber**	**455 Calories**	**3**
3	1	3	80	1
7	16	2	190	-
0	0	3	60	1
10 g Protein	**17 g Fat**	**8 g Fiber**	**330 Calories**	**2**
28	3	0	140	-
0	0	0	20	-
9	0	6	320	3
0	0	1	20	-
1	0	1.5	12.5	-
1	0	1.5	12.5	-
7	8	0	100	-
7	2	7	120	1
53 g Protein	**13 g Fat**	**17 g Fiber**	**745 Calories**	**4**
4	0	4	90	1
0	10	0	90	-
4 g Protein	**10 g Fat**	**4 g Fiber**	**180 Calories**	**1**
121 g Protein	**62.5 g Fat**	**50 g Fiber**	**2345 Calories**	**16**
22%	**25%**			

MEAL	FOOD ITEM	SERVING SIZE	GRAMS OF CARBOHYDRATE
Breakfast			
	Smoothie:		
	Soy milk, unflavored	8 fluid ounces	8
	Blueberries, frozen	¾ cup	15
	Nonfat greek yogurt (plain)	6 ounces	13
	Banana	1, small	15
	Mango, cubes	½ cup	15
	Ground flaxseed meal	2 tablespoons	4
			70 g Carb
Morning snack			
	Apple	1, small	15
			15 g Carb
Lunch			
	Thin-crust cheese pizza	¼ of 12 inch pie	30
	Beans	½ cup	15
	Salad greens	2 cups	10
	Sliced tomatoes	½ cup	2.5
	Dried cranberries	1 tablespoon	7
	Sunflower seeds	4 tablespoons	8
	Sliced carrots	½ cup	2.5
	Salad dressing	2 tablespoons	0
			75 g Carb
Afternoon snack			
	String cheese	2 (one-ounce) sticks	0
	Tangerine	2, small	15
			15 g Carb
Dinner			
	Salmon (herb seasoning)	4 ounces	0
	Olive oil	1 tablespoon	0
	Roasted carrots	½ cup	5
	Roasted brussels sprouts	½ cup	5
	Brown rice	1 cup	45
			55 g Carb
Evening snack			
	Low-fat cottage cheese, herb flavored	1 cup	6
	Multigrain crackers	10	30
			36 g Carb
		TOTALS	**265 g Carb**
			45%

GRAMS OF PROTEIN	GRAMS OF FAT	GRAMS OF FIBER	TOTAL CALORIES	# OF CARB "CHOICES"
6	4	1	90	½
0	0	3	60	1
16	0	0	120	1
0	0	3	60	1
0	0	3	60	1
3	6	4	80	-
25 g Protein	**10 g Fat**	**14 g Fiber**	**470 Calories**	**4.5**
0	0	3	60	1
		3 g Fiber	**60 Calories**	**1**
10	7.5	0	178	1
8	1	8	115	1
4	0	5	50	1
1	0	1	12	-
0	0	-	30	½
6	16	2	180	-
1	0	1	12	-
0	10	0	90	-
30 g Protein	**34.5 g Fat**	**18 g Fiber**	**697 Calories**	**3.5**
16	10	0	160	-
0	0	3	60	1
16 g Protein	**10 g Fat**	**3 g Fiber**	**220 Calories**	**1**
28	12	0	220	-
0	12	0	120	-
2	0	3	25	-
2	0	3	25	-
6	2	4	215	3
38 g Protein	**26 g Fat**	**10 g Fiber**	**605 Calories**	**3**
28	2	0	160	-
6	0	4	160	2
34 g Protein	**2 g Fat**	**4 g Fiber**	**320 Calories**	**2**
143 g Protein	**82.5 g Fat**	**52 g Fiber**	**2372 Calories**	**15**
24%	**31%**			

Appendix 2: Food Journal

Keeping a food journal is a scientifically proven way to stay attuned to how you're eating and help you stick with your goals. Try making a commitment to track the times you eat or drink, what you had, how much, the grams of carb per portion, and how hungry you were on a scale of 1 to 10 (1 being "not hungry," 10 being "starved"). Remember, eating when your hunger is a 5 or 6 increases the odds of being able to control your portions.

DATE/ TIME	FOOD/BEVERAGE CONSUMED	AMOUNT EATEN	GRAMS OF CARBS	HUNGER SCALE (1–10)

Resources

Diabetes and Prediabetes

Complete Guide to Carb Counting: How to Take the Mystery Out of Carb Counting and Improve Your Blood Glucose Control, by Hope S. Warshaw and Karmeen Kulkarni (Alexandria, VA: American Diabetes Association, 2011)

Diabetes Weight Loss Week by Week: A Safe, Effective Method for Losing Weight and Improving Your Health, by Jill Weisenberger (Alexandria, VA: American Diabetes Association, 2012)

Eat What You Love, Love What You Eat with Diabetes: A Mindful Eating Program for Thriving with Prediabetes or Diabetes, by Megrette Fletcher and Michelle May (Oakland, CA: New Harbinger Publications, 2012)

The Everything Guide to Managing and Reversing Pre-diabetes, by Gretchen Scalpi (Avon, MA: Adams Media, 2010)

"Glycemic Index and Glycemic Load for 100+ Foods"
www.health.harvard.edu/newsweek/Glycemic_index_and_glycemic_load_for_100_foods.htm
Provides information about how foods affect blood sugar and insulin. The lower a food's glycemic index or glycemic load, the less it affects blood sugar and insulin levels.

Dining Out

Eat Out Healthy, by Joanne "Dr. Jo" Lichten (Fort Lauderdale, FL: Nutrifit Publishing, 2012)

What to Eat When You're Eating Out: What to Eat in America's Most Popular Chain Restaurants, by Hope Warshaw (Alexandria, VA: Small Steps Press, American Diabetes Association, 2009)

Mindful Eating

Intuitive Eating: A Revolutionary Program That Works, 3rd edition, by Evelyn Tribole and Elyse Resch (New York: St. Martin's Griffin, 2012)

Center for Mindful Eating

www.tcme.org

A forum for people interested in developing, deepening, and understanding the value and importance of mindful eating.

General Nutrition and Healthy Eating

Cholesterol Down: 10 Simple Steps to Lower Your cholesterol in 4 Weeks—Without Prescription Drugs, by Janet Brill (New York: Crown/Three Rivers Press, 2006)

The DASH Diet Action Plan: Proven to Boost Weight Loss and Improve Health, by Marla Heller (New York: Grand Central Life & Style, 2011)

101 Foods That Could Save Your Life, by David W. Grotto (New York: Bantam, 2010)

Center for Science in the Public Interest

www.cspinet.org

Award-winning website of the *Nutrition Action Healthletter*, a terrific resource for keeping up on what is happening in the field of nutrition and health.

ChooseMyPlate, US Department of Agriculture

www.ChooseMyPlate.gov

Offers numerous free tools to help you plan, analyze, and track your diet and physical activity.

Cooking Light

www.cookinglight.com

The website of the highly respected *Cooking Light* magazine provides thousands of free recipes tested by professionals and registered dietitians to meet stringent nutritional requirements and high flavor standards.

Eating Well

www.eatingwell.com

The website of *Eating Well* magazine provides thousands of beautifully presented and healthful recipes.

Eat Right: Academy of Nutrition and Dietetics

www.eatright.org

This public information center provides extensive food and nutrition resources for consumers.

Epicurious

www.epicurious.com/recipesmenus/healthy/recipes

The healthy recipes section of Epicurious.com—a website dedicated to recipes, cooking, drinking, entertaining, and restaurants—offers some great choices.

Fruits & Veggies: More Matters

www.fruitsandveggiesmorematters.org

Great resource for learning how to incorporate more fruits and vegetables into your diet. Full of practical tips.

World's Healthiest Foods

www.whfoods.com

This foodie website offers extensive information on the benefits of eating healthy foods, along with a comprehensive database describing the nutritional benefits of hundreds of foods and how to select, store, and prepare them. Also provides scientific study citations to support information.

Tools for Tracking Food, Activity, and Goals

Calorie King

www.calorieking.com

Comprehensive website with a food database containing nutritional information for most American generic and brand-name foods.

Endomondo

www.endomondo.com

Track your workouts and set up exercise challenges with other connected friends. Apps available for Apple, Android, and Blackberry smartphones.

Fooducate: Eat a Bit Better

www.fooducate.com

Offers a smartphone app for scanning food bar codes that rates foods and indicates healthier alternatives.

Good Measures

www.goodmeasures.com

Good Measures is a web and smartphone-based nutrition system that allows users to track food and physical activity and receive real-time feedback on how to best meet their nutrition and health goals.

Lose It!

www.loseit.com

Apple and Android smartphone app that tracks calories and exercise, allowing users to set up individualized weight-loss plans.

My Fitness Pal

www.myfitnesspal.com

Website and app (for Apple and Android smartphones) for tracking food and activity. Members can connect with each other to form a "fitness community."

Nutrition Facts and Calorie Counter

www.nutritiondata.com

Provides complete nutrition information for foods and helps you select foods that best match your dietary needs. Offers a smartphone app as well.

Reference Websites

Consumer Lab

www.consumerlab.com

A terrific resource for deciding on quality dietary supplement and herbal products. The Consumer Lab tests and reviews a variety of supplements, reports findings on content and quality, and then rates them as approved or disapproved for use. Small annual fee required.

Glycemic Index and International GI Database

www.glycemicindex.com

The official website of the glycemic index and GI database, which is based in the Human Nutrition Unit, School of Molecular Biosciences, at the University of Sydney.

Notes

Introduction

1. National Diabetes Education Program, "The Link Between Diabetes and Cardiovascular Disease," February 2007, online at http://ndep.nih.gov/media/CVD_FactSheet.pdf.
2. F. B. Hu, J. E. Manson, M. J. Stampfer, G. Colditz, S. Liu, C. G. Solomon, and W. C. Willett, "Diet, Lifestyle, and the Risk of Type 2 Diabetes Mellitus in Women," *New England Journal of Medicine* 345, no. 11 (2001): 790–97, online at www.ncbi.nlm.nih.gov/pubmed/11556298?dopt=. This is also known as the Harvard Nurse's Health study.
3. Standards of Medical Care in Diabetes–2013, American Diabetes Association http://care.diabetesjournals.org/content/36/Supplement_1/S11.full.

Chapter 1

1. "National Diabetes Prevention Program Summary," Centers for Disease Control, 2012, online at www.cdc.gov/diabetes/prevention/newsroom/overview.htm.
2. David M. Nathan, Mayer B. Davidson, Ralph A. DeFronzo, Robert J. Heine, Robert R. Henry, Richard Pratley, and Bernard Zinman, "Impaired Fasting Glucose and Impaired Glucose Tolerance Implications for Care," *Diabetes Care* 30, no. 3 (March 2007): 753–59, online at http://m.care.diabetesjournals.org/content/30/3/753.full.
3. "Diabetes Statistics," data from the 2011 National Diabetes Fact Sheet (released January 26, 2011), online at www.diabetes.org/diabetes-basics/diabetes-statistics.
4. "Number (in Millions) of Civilian, Noninstitutionalized Persons with Diagnosed Diabetes, United States, 1980–2011." Centers for Disease Control, online at www.cdc.gov/diabetes/Statistics/prev/national/figpersons.htm.
5. "Prediabetes Among People Aged 20 Years or Older, United States, 2010," data from the 2011 National Diabetes Fact Sheet, online at www.cdc.gov/diabetes/pubs/estimates11.htm#7.
6. "Nutrition and the Health of Young People," Centers for Disease Control, online at www.cdc.gov/HealthyYouth/Nutrition/pdf/facts.pdf.
7. William H. Herman, "The Economic Costs of Diabetes," *Diabetes Care* 36, no. 4 (April 2013): 1033–46.
8. "National Defense Budget Estimates for FY 2012," Office of the Undersecretary of Defense, March 2011, online at http://comptroller.defense.gov/defbudget/fy2012/FY12_Green_Book.pdf.
9. "Number of Americans with Diabetes Projected to Double or Triple by 2050," press release, October 22, 2010, online at www.cdc.gov/media/pressrel/2010/r101022.html.
10. "Genetics and Diabetes: What's Your Risk?" Joslin Diabetes Center, online at www.joslin.org/info/genetics_and_diabetes.html.
11. Gerald Reaven, "Insulin Resistance: A Chicken That Has Come to Roost," *Annals of the New York Academy of Sciences*, 892 (November 1999): 45–57.
12. "Simple Steps to Preventing Diabetes," Harvard School of Public Health, online at www.hsph.harvard.edu/nutritionsource/diabetes-prevention/preventing-diabetes-full-story/index.html.

13. F. B. Hu, J. E. Manson, M. J. Stampfer, G. Colditz, S. Liu, C. G. Solomon, and W. C. Willett, "Diet, Lifestyle, and the Risk of Type 2 Diabetes Mellitus in Women," *New England Journal of Medicine* 345, no. 11 (2001): 790–97, online at www.ncbi.nlm.nih.gov/pubmed/11556298?dopt=.

14. D. Mozaffarian, "Lifestyle Risk Factors and New-Onset Diabetes Mellitus in Older Adults: The Cardiovascular Health Study," *Archives of Internal Medicine* 169, no. 8 (2009): 798–807.

15. "Diabetes Overview," US Department of Health and Human Services, National Institute of Diabetes and Digestive and Kidney Diseases (NIDDK), online at http://diabetes.niddk.nih.gov/dm/pubs/overview.

16. Mitchell A. Lazar, "How Obesity Causes Cancer: Not a Tall Tale," online at www.med.upenn.edu/lazarlab/Pubs_pdf/lazar%20science_2005.pdf.

17. G. Hu, "Physical Activity, Body Mass Index, and Risk of Type 2 Diabetes in Patients with Normal or Impaired Glucose Regulation," *Archives of Internal Medicine* 164 (April 26, 2004): 892–6.

18. C. Y. Jeon, "Physical Activity of Moderate Intensity and Risk of Type 2 Diabetes," *Diabetes Care* 30, no. 3 (March 2007): 744–52.

19. Ibid.

20. Hsin-Chieh Yeh, "Smoking, Smoking Cessation, and Risk for Type 2 Diabetes Mellitus," *Annals of Internal Medicine* 152, no. 1 (January 2010):10–17.

21. L. A. Bazzano, "Prevention of Type 2 Diabetes by Diet and Lifestyle Modification," *Journal of the American College of Nutrition* 24, no. 5 (2005): 310–19.

22. Ibid.

23. www.diabetes.org/food-and-fitness/food/what-can-I-eat-carbohydrates.html.

24. "What Is the Effect of Saturated Fat Intake on Increased Risk of Cardiovascular Disease or Type 2 Diabetes?" USDA Nutrition Evidence Library, online at www.nutritionevidencelibrary.com/evidence.cfm?evidence_summary_id=250189.

25. Haitao Wen, Denis Gris, Yu Lei, Sushmita Jha, Lu Zhang, Max Tze-Han Huang, Willie June Brickey, and Jenny P-Y Ting, "Fatty Acid–Induced NLRP3-ASC Inflammasome Activation Interferes with Insulin Signaling," *Nature Immunology*, online at www.nature.com/ni/journal/v12/n5/full/ni.2022.html.

26. V. S. Malik, "Sugar-Sweetened Beverages and Risk of Metabolic Syndrome and Type 2 Diabetes: A Meta-Analysis," *Diabetes Care* 33, no. 11 (November 2010): 2477–83.

27. Lawrence de Koning, Vasanti S. Malik, Eric B. Rimm, Walter C. Willett, and Frank B. Hu, "Sugar-Sweetened and Artificially Sweetened Beverage Consumption and Risk of Type 2 Diabetes in Men," *American Journal of Clinical Nutrition* 93, no. 6 (June 2011): 1321–27, online at www.ajcn.org/content/93/6/1321.full.pdf+html.

28. Ibid.

29. Charles M. Alexander, Pamela B. Landsman, Steven M. Teutsch, and Steven M. Haffner, "NCEP-Defined Metabolic Syndrome, Diabetes, and Prevalence of Coronary Heart Disease Among NHANES III Participants Age 50 Years and Older," *Diabetes* 52, no. 5 (May 2003): 1210–14, online at http://diabetes.diabetesjournals.org/content/52/5/1210.full.

30. "About Metabolic Syndrome," American Heart Association, online at www.heart.org/HEARTORG/Conditions/More/MetabolicSyndrome/About-Metabolic-Syndrome_UCM_301920_Article.jsp.

31. *Third Report of the National cholesterol Education Program (NCEP)*, online at www.nhlbi.nih.gov/cgibin/search?q=cache:M6yAVuqvaj0J:www.nhlbi.nih.gov/ guidelines/cholesterol/atp3full.pdf+waist+hip+ratio+metabolic+syndrome+&site= NHLBI_Public&client=NHLBI_Public_frontend&proxystylesheet=NHLBI_Public_ frontend&output=xml_no_dtd&oe=ISO-8859-1&ie=ISO-8859-1&access=p.

32. Scott M. Grundy, "Does a Diagnosis of Metabolic Syndrome Have Value in Clinical Practice?" *American Journal of Clinical Nutrition* 83, no. 6 (June 2006): 1248–51, online at www.ajcn.org/content/83/6/1248.full.

33. S. Mottillo, "The Metabolic Syndrome and Cardiovascular Risk: A Systemic Review and Meta-analysis," *Journal of the American College of Cardiology* 56, no. 14 (September 2010): 1113–32, online at www.ncbi.nlm.nih.gov/pubmed/20863953.

34. "Who Is at Risk for Metabolic Syndrome?," National Heart, Lung, and Blood Institute, online at www.nhlbi.nih.gov/health/health-topics/topics/ms/atrisk.html.

35. "What About Diabetes in Asian Americans? Am I at Risk?" Joslin Diabetes Center, online at http://aadi.joslin.org/content/diabetes-asians-asian-americans.

36. Chee-Eng Tan, Stefan Ma, Daniel Wai, Suok-Kai Chew, and E.-Shyong Tai, "Can We Apply the National Cholesterol Education Program Adult Treatment Panel Definition of the Metabolic Syndrome to Asians?" *Diabetes Care* 27, no. 5 (May 2004): 1182–86, online at http://care.diabetesjournals.org/content/27/5/1182.full.pdf+html.

37. "Why Do People of Asian Decent Get Diabetes?" Joslin Diabetes Center, online at http://aadi.joslin.org/content/asian/why-are-asians-higher-risk-diabetes.

38. "Does PCOS Put Women at Risk for Other Health Problems?" US Dept. of Health and Human Services Office on Women's Health, data from Polycystic Ovary Syndrome Fact Sheet, online at www.womenshealth.gov/publications/our-publications/fact-sheet/ polycystic-ovary-syndrome.cfm#j.

39. Helen Mason, "Polycystic Ovary Syndrome (PCOS) Trilogy: A Translation and Clinical Review," *Clinical Endocrinology* 69, no. 6 (2008): 831–44.

40. S. Grundy, "Prediabetes, Metabolic Syndrome, and Cardiovascular Risk," *Journal of the American College of Cardiology* 59, no. 7 (2012): 635–43; and S. Milman, J. Crandall, et al., "Mechanisms of Vascular Complications in Prediabetes," *Medical Clinics of North America* 95, no. 2 (March 2011): 309–25, vii.

41. S. Oriz-Filho et al., "(Pre)diabetes, Brain, Aging, and Cognition," *Biochimica et Biophysica Acta* 1792, no. 5 (May 2009): 432–43, online at www.ncbi.nlm.nih.gov/pubmed/19135149.

42. B. Arcidiacono, "Insulin Resistance and Cancer Risk: An Overview of the Pathogenetic Mechanisms," *Experimental Diabetes Research* Vol. 2012: 1–12, online at www.ncbi.nlm. nih.gov/pmc/articles/PMC3372318.

43. E. Giovannucci, "Diabetes and Cancer: A Consensus Report," *Diabetes Care* 33, no. 7 (July 2010): 1674–85.

44. Dariush Mozaffarian, Aruna Kamineni, Mercedes Carnethon, Luc Djoussé, Kenneth J. Mukamal, and David Siscovick, "Lifestyle Risk Factors and New-Onset Diabetes Mellitus in Older Adults: The Cardiovascular Health Study," *Archives of Internal Medicine* 169, no. 8 (2009): 798–807, online at http://archinte.jamanetwork.com/article.aspx?volume= 169&issue=8&page=798#ref-ioi80218-2; and "Lifestyle Factors Related to Risk of Diabetes Among Older Adults," *Medical News Today*, April 29, 2009, online at www.medicalnewstoday.com/releases/148008.php.

45. "Guidelines for Diabetes Mellitus Management: Standards of Medical Care," American Diabetes Association, 2013, online at http://care.diabetesjournals.org/content/36/Supplement_1/S11.full.

Chapter 2

1. Gerald Reaven, "Insulin Resistance: A Chicken That Has Come to Roost," *Annals of the New York Academy of Sciences* 892 (November 1999): 45–57.
2. "Living with Diabetes: What Is a Normal Non fasting Blood Sugar Level?" American Diabetes Association, online at www.diabetes.org/living-with-diabetes/treatment-and-care/ask-the-expert/ask-the-pharmacist/archives/what-is-a-normal-non-fasting.html.
3. "Insulin Resistance and Prediabetes," National Diabetes Information Clearing House, online at http://diabetes.niddk.nih.gov/DM/pubs/insulinresistance.
4. Ibid.
5. Eric Westman, "Is Dietary Carbohydrate Essential for Human Health?" *American Journal of Clinical Nutrition* 75, no. 5 (May 2002): 951–53.
6. Gerald Reaven, "The Metabolic Syndrome. Is a Diagnosis Necessary?" *American Journal of Clinical Nutrition* 84, no. 5 (November 2006): 1237–47.
7. W. C. Knowler, "Reduction in the Incidence of Type 2 Diabetes with Lifestyle Intervention or Metformin," *New England Journal of Medicine* 346, no. 6 (February 7, 2002): 393–403.
8. The findings of the Finnish Diabetes Prevention Study are published in J. Tuomilehto, "Prevention of Type 2 Diabetes Mellitus by Changes in Lifestyle Among Subjects with Impaired Glucose Tolerance," *New England Journal of Medicine* 344, no. 18 (May 3, 2001): 1343–50.
9. The findings of the Diabetes Prevention Program are published in W. Knowler et al., "Reduction in the Incidence of Type 2 Diabetes with Lifestyle Intervention or Metformin," *New England Journal of Medicine* 346, no. 6 (February 7, 2002): 393–403.
10. L. Perrault, "Effect of Regression from Prediabetes to Normal Glucose Regulation on Long-Term Reduction in Diabetes Risk: Results from the Diabetes Prevention Program Outcomes Study," *Lancet* 379, no. 9833 (June 16, 2012): 2243–51.
11. Diabetes Prevention Program Research Group, "Ten-Year Follow-Up of Diabetes Incidence and Weight Loss in the Diabetes Prevention Program Outcomes Study," *Lancet* 374, no. 9702 (November 14, 2009): 1677–86.
12. T. J. Orchard, "Long-Term Effects of the Diabetes Prevention Program Interventions on Cardiovascular Risk Factors: A Report from the DPP Outcomes Study," *Diabetic Medicine* 30, no. 1 (January 2013): 46–55.

Chapter 3

1. "What We Eat in America: NHANES 2009-2010, National Health and Examination Survey," National Center for Health Statistics, Centers for Disease Control.
2. Hodan Farah Wells and Jean C. Buzby, "Dietary Assessment of Major Trends in US Food Consumption, 1970–2005," US Department of Agriculture, online at www.ers.usda.gov/media/210681/eib33_1_.pdf.
3. R. Johnson, "Dietary Sugar Intake and Cardiovascular Health: A Scientific Statement from the American Heart Association," *Circulation* 120 (2009): 1011–20.
4. J. Welsh, Andrea J. Sharma, Lisa Grellinger, and Miriam B. Vos, "Consumption of Added Sugars Is Decreasing in the United States," *American Journal of Clinical Nutrition* 94, no. 3 (September 2011): 726–34, online at http://ajcn.nutrition.org/content/94/3/726.abstract.

5. "Dietary Guidelines for Americans," 2010, US Department of Agriculture, US Department of Health and Human Services, online at www.cnpp.usda.gov/publications/dietaryguidelines/2010/policydoc/policydoc.pdf.

6. R. Post, "Dietary Fiber for the Treatment of Type 2 Diabetes Mellitus: A Meta-analysis," *Journal of the American Board of Family Medicine* 25, no. 1 (January–February 2012): 16–23.

7. E. Theuwissen and R. P. Mensink, "Water Soluble Dietary Fibers and Cardiovascular Disease," *Physiology and Behavior* 94, no. 2 (May 2008): 285–92, online at www.ncbi.nlm.nih.gov/pubmed/18302966.

Chapter 4

1. "The New American Plate," American Institute for Cancer Research, online at www.aicr.org/new-american-plate; and "Healthy Eating Plate," Harvard School of Public Health, online at www.hsph.harvard.edu/nutritionsource/healthy-eating-plate.

Chapter 5

1. "SuperTracker," US Department of Agriculture, online at https://www.choosemyplate.gov/SuperTracker.

2. "Calorie Counter Calculator," American Cancer Society, online at www.cancer.org/healthy/toolsandcalculators/calculators/app/calorie-counter-calculator.

3. "Adult Weight Management Determination of Resting Metabolic Rate," Academy of Nutrition and Dietetics Evidence Analysis Library, online at www.adaevidencelibrary.com/template.cfm?template=guide_summary&key=621; and Mark D. Muffin, Sachiko T. St. Jeor, et al., "A New Predictive Equation for Resting Energy Expenditure in Healthy Individuals," *American Journal of Clinical Nutrition* 51, no. 2 (February 1990): 241–47, online at www.ajcn.org/content/51/2/241.long; and J. R. Dobratz, S. D. Sibley, T. R. Beckman, B. J. Valentine, T. A. Kellogg, S. Ikramuddin, and C. P. Earthman, "Predicting Energy Expenditure in Extremely Obese Women," *Journal of Parenteral and Enteral Nutrition* 31, no. 3 (May–June 2007): 217–27, online at www.ncbi.nlm.nih.gov/pubmed/17463148.

4. "Human Energy Requirements: Report of a Joint FAO/WHO/UNU Expert Consultation Rome," October 17–24, 2001, online at ftp://ftp.fao.org/docrep/fao/007/y5686e/y5686e00.pdf.

5. Brian Wansink, *Mindless Eating: Why We Eat More Than We Think* (New York: Bantam, 2007).

6. Richard J. Schrot, "Targeting Plasma Glucose: Preprandial Versus Postprandial," *Clinical Diabetes* 22, no. 4 (October 2004): 169–72, online at http://clinical.diabetesjournals.org/content/22/4/169.full.pdf+html.

7. "Choose Your Foods: Exchange Lists for Diabetes," American Diabetes Association, online at www.shopdiabetes.org/176-Choose-Your-Foods-Exchange-Lists-for-Diabetes-Singles.aspx.

Chapter 6

1. "Choose Your Foods: Exchange Lists for Diabetes," American Diabetes Association, online at www.shopdiabetes.org/176-Choose-Your-Foods-Exchange-Lists-for-Diabetes-Singles.aspx.

2. B. Farmer, B. T. Larson, V. L. Fulgoni 3rd, A. J. Rainville, and G. U. Liepa, "A Vegetarian Dietary Pattern as a Nutrient-Dense Approach to Weight Management: An Analysis of the National Health and Nutrition Examination Survey, 1999–2004," *Journal of the American Dietetic Association* 111, no. 6 (June 2011): 819–27, online at www.ncbi.nlm.nih .gov/pubmed/21616194.

3. "Carbohydrates," American Diabetes Association, online at www.diabetes.org/ food-and-fitness/food/what-can-i-eat/carbohydrates.html.

4. "Choose Your Foods. Exchange Lists for Diabetes," American Diabetes Association and American Dietetic Association, online at http://www.shopdiabetes.org/ 176-Choose-Your-Foods-Exchange-Lists-for-Diabetes-Singles.aspx.

Chapter 7

1. M. Garaulet, P. Gómez-Abellán, J. J. Alburquerque-Béjar, Y. C. Lee, J. M. Ordovás, and F. A. Scheer, "Timing of Food Intake Predicts Weight Loss Effectiveness," *International Journal of Obesity* (London) (January 29, 2013), online at www.ncbi.nlm.nih.gov/ pubmed?term=international%20journal%20of%20obesity%20scheer.

2. Ibid.

Chapter 8

1. "Nutrition Recommendations and Interventions for Diabetes: A Position Statement of the American Diabetes Association," *Diabetes Care*, online at http://care.diabetesjournals.org/ content/31/Supplement_1/S61.long.

2. "Diabetes Mellitus in Adults: Standards of Medical Care, 2012," American Diabetes Association, online at http://care.diabetesjournals.org/content/35/Supplement_1/ S11.extract.

3. Cara B. Ebbeling, Michael M. Leidig, Henry A. Feldman, Margaret M. Lovesky, and David S. Ludwig, "Effects of a Low Glycemic Load vs. Low Fat Diet in Obese Young Adults: A Randomized Trial," *Journal of the American Medical Association* 297, no. 19 (2007): 2092–102, online at http://jama.jamanetwork.com/article.aspx?articleid=207088.

4. L. G. Ogden et al., "Cluster Analysis of the National Weight Control Registry to Identify Distinct Subgroups Maintaining Successful Weight Loss," *Obesity* (April 3, 2012), doi: 10.1038/oby.2012.79.

5. S. Phelan, "Are the Eating and Exercise Habits of Successful Weight Losers Changing?" *Obesity* 14 (2006): 710–16.

6. Rena R. Wing , Deborah F. Tate, Amy A. Gorin, Hollie A. Raynor, and Joseph L. Fava, "A Self-Regulation Program for Maintenance of Weight Loss," *New England Journal of Medicine* 355 (2006): 1563–71, online at www.nejm.org/doi/pdf/10.1056/NEJMoa061883.

7. F. M. Sacks, "Comparison of Weight-Loss Diets with Different Compositions of Fat, Protein, and Carbohydrates," *New England Journal of Medicine* 360, no. 9 (February 2009): 859–73.

8. D. Paddon-Jones, "Protein, Weight Management, and Satiety," *American Journal of Clinical Nutrition* 87 (May 2008): 1558S–1561S.

9. D. K. Layman, "A Reduced Ratio of Dietary Carbohydrate to Protein Improves Body Composition and Blood Lipid Profiles During Weight Loss in Adult Women," *Journal of Nutrition* 133 (February 2003): 411–17.

10. M. Garaulet, "Timing of Food Intake Predicts Weight Loss Effectiveness," *International Journal of Obesity* 37 (April 2013): 604–611, online at www.nature.com/ijo/journal/v37/n4/full/ijo2012229a.html.
11. James Prochaska, *Changing for Good* (New York: William Morrow, 2007); and "Detailed Overview of the Transtheoretical Model," Cancer Prevention Research Center, online at www.uri.edu/research/cprc/TTM/detailedoverview.htm.

Chapter 9

1. Data from the 2011 National Diabetes Fact Sheet (released January 26, 2011), American Diabetes Association, online at www.diabetes.org/diabetes-basics/diabetes-statistics.
2. "About Metabolic Syndrome," American Heart Association, online at www.heart.org/HEARTORG/Conditions/More/MetabolicSyndrome/About-Metabolic-Syndrome_UCM_301920_Article.jsp.
3. "What Your cholesterol Levels Mean," American Heart Association, online at www.heart.org/HEARTORG/Conditions/cholesterol/Aboutcholesterol/What-Your-cholesterol-Levels-Mean_UCM_305562_Article.jsp.
4. "Understanding Blood Pressure Readings," American Heart Association, online at www.heart.org/HEARTORG/Conditions/HighBloodPressure/AboutHighBloodPressure/Understanding-Blood-Pressure-Readings_UCM_301764_Article.jsp.
5. "Prediabetes Facts," American Diabetes Association, online at www.diabetes.org/diabetes-basics/prevention/pre-diabetes/pre-diabetes-faqs.html.
6. "Your Guide to Lowering Your Blood Pressure with DASH," National Heart, Lung, and Blood Institute, online at www.nhlbi.nih.gov/health/public/heart/hbp/dash/new_dash.pdf.

Chapter 10

1. V. A. Hughes, "Exercise Increases Muscle GLUT-4 Levels and Insulin Action in Subjects with Impaired Glucose Tolerance," *American Journal of Physiology* 264, no. 6 (part 1) (June 1993): E855–62.
2. S. A. Dugan et al., "Physical Activity and Reduced Intra-Abdominal Fat in Midlife African American and White Women," *Obesity* 18, no. 6 (June 2010): 1260–65.
3. "Physical Activity and Health: A Report of the Surgeon General," CDC, online at www.cdc.gov/NCCDPHP/SGR/summ.htm.
4. J. Tuomilehto, "Nonpharmacologic Therapy and Exercise in the Prevention of Type 2 Diabetes," *Diabetes Care* 32 suppl. 2 (November 2009): S 189–93.
5. Stephen K. Malin, Robert Gerber, Stuart R. Chipkin, and Barry Braun, "Independent and Combined Effects of Exercise Training and Metformin on Insulin Sensitivity in Individuals with Prediabetes," *Diabetes Care* 35, no. 1 (January 2012): 131–36, online at http://care.diabetesjournals.org/content/35/1/131.long.
6. F. Orio, "Metabolic and Cardiopulmonary Effect of Detraining After a Structured Exercise Training Programme in Young PCOS Women," *Clinical Endocrinology* 68 (2008): 976–81.
7. N. King, "Beneficial Effects of Exercise: Shifting the Focus from Body Weight to Other Markers of Health," *British Journal of Sports Medicine*, September 29, 2009, online at www.ncbi.nlm.nih.gov/pubmed/?term=Beneficial+Effects+Of+of+Exercise%3A+Shifting+The+the+Focus+From+from+Body+Weight+To+to+Other+Markers+Of+of+Health.

8. "Physical Activity and Public Health: Updated Recommendation for Adults from Guidelines," American College of Sports Medicine and the American Heart Association, *Circulation* 116 (2007): 1081–93, online at http://circ.ahajournals.org/content/116/9/1081.full.pdf.

9. "Physical Activity Guidelines for Americans," US Department of Health and Human Services, online at www.health.gov/paguidelines.

Chapter 11

1 Jia-Yi Dong, "Magnesium Intake and Risk of Type 2 Diabetes: Meta-analysis of Prospective Cohort Studies," *Diabetes Care* 34, no. 9 (September 2011): 2116–22, online at www.ncbi.nlm.nih.gov/pmc/articles/PMC3161260.

2. "Institute of Medicine Dietary Reference Intakes (DRIs)," Food and Nutrition Board, Institute of Medicine, National Academies, online at http://iom.edu/Activities/Nutrition/SummaryDRIs/~/media/Files/Activity%20Files/Nutrition/DRIs/RDA%20and%20AIs_Vitamin%20and%20Elements.pdf.

3. "Dietary Fact Sheet: Magnesium," National Institutes of Health, online at http.//ods.od.nih.gov/factsheets/Magnesium-HealthProfessional.

4. A. A. Ginde, "Demographic Differences and Trends of Vitamin D Insufficiency in the US Population, 1988–2004," *Archives of Internal Medicine* 169, no. 6 (March 23, 2009): 626–32.

5. R. Zhang, "Vitamin D in Health and Disease: Current Perspectives," *Nutrition Journal* 9 (December 8, 2010): 65, online at www.ncbi.nlm.nih.gov/pmc/articles/PMC3019131.

6. M. F. Holick, "Vitamin D: A D-Lightful Health Perspective," *Nutrition Review* 66, no. 10 (suppl 2) (October 2008): S182–94, online at www.ncbi.nlm.nih.gov/pubmed?term=Vitamin%20D%3A%20a%20D-Lightful%20helath%20perspective%20holick.

7. Chih-Chien Sung, Min-Tser Liao, Kuo-Cheng Lu, and Chia-Chao Wu, "Role of Vitamin D in Insulin Resistance," *Journal of Biomedicine and Biotechnology* (2012), online only at www.ncbi.nlm.nih.gov/pmc/articles/PMC3440067.

8. Nishan S. Kalupahana, Kate J. Claycombe, and Naima Moustaid-Moussa, "(n-3) Fatty Acids Alleviate Adipose Tissue Inflammation and Insulin Resistance: Mechanistic Insights," *Advances in Nutrition* 2, no. 4 (July 2011): 304–16, online at www.ncbi.nlm.nih.gov/pmc/articles/PMC3125680.

9. "Natural Medicines Comprehensive Database: Scientific Gold Standard for Evidence-Based, Clinical Information on Natural Medicines," October 2012, www.naturaldatabase.com.

10. "Dietary Reference Intakes (DRIs)," Food and Nutrition Board, Institute of Medicine, National Academies, online at http://iom.edu/Activities/Nutrition/SummaryDRIs/~/media/Files/Activity%20Files/Nutrition/DRIs/RDA%20and%20AIs_Vitamin%20and%20Elements.pdf.

11. "Chromium Toxicity: What Is Chromium?," Agency for Toxic Substances and Disease Registry (ATSDR), US Department of Health and Human Services, online at www.atsdr.cdc.gov/csem/csem.asp?csem=10&po=4.

12. M. J. Leach and S. Kumar, "Cinnamon for Diabetes Mellitus," *Cochrane Database of Systematic Reviews*, September 12, 2012, online at www.ncbi.nlm.nih.gov/pubmed/22972104; and T. Lu, H. Sheng, J. Wu, Y. Cheng, J. Zhu, and Y. Chen, "Cinnamon Extract Improves Fasting Blood Glucose and Glycosylated Hemoglobin Level in Chinese Patients with Type 2 Diabetes," *Nutrition Research* 32, no. 6 (June 2012): 408–12.

Chapter 12

1. "How to Understand and Use the Nutrition Facts Label," Food and Drug Administration, online at www.fda.gov/Food/ResourcesForYou/Consumers/NFLPM/ucm274593.htm.
2. "Food Nutrition, Physical Activity, and the Prevention of Cancer: A Global Perspective—Animal Foods," American Institute for Cancer Research, online at www.dietandcancerreport.org/expert_report/recommendations/recommendation_animal_foods.php.

About the Author

Hillary Wright is a registered and licensed dietitian with more than two decades of experience counseling clients on diet and lifestyle change. She holds a bachelor's degree in human nutrition from the University of Massachusetts at Amherst and a master's of education in health education from Boston University.

Hillary is the director of nutrition counseling for the Domar Center for Mind/Body Health in Waltham, Massachusetts, where she specializes in diabetes prevention and women's health issues. She is the author of *The PCOS Diet Plan: A Natural Approach to Health for Women with Polycystic Ovary Syndrome.*

She is also a nutrition writer, speaker, and consultant to industry and health-related organizations, including the nutrition logging system GoodMeasures.com, and has been quoted widely in national media. She holds a part-time position as a nutritionist for the Dana Farber CancerInstitute in Boston, counseling patients during cancer treatment as well as cancer survivors through the Adult Survivorship Clinic. Visit www.prediabetesdietbook.com.

Index

Also by Hillary Wright

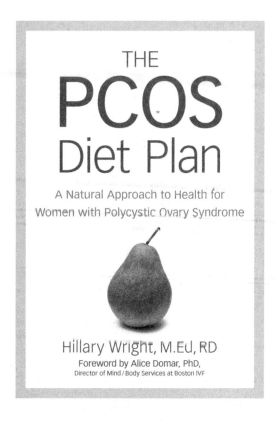

The PCOS Diet Plan
A Natural Approach to Health for
Women with Polycystic Ovary Syndrome

$18.99 paperback (Canada: $20.99)

ISBN: 978-1-58761-023-3
eBook ISBN: 978-1-58761-364-7

Available from Ten Speed Press wherever books are sold.